IN THE COMPANY OF MY SISTERS

MY STORY, MY TRUTH

KAREN EUBANKS JACKSON

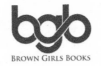

BROWN GIRLS BOOKS

CONTENTS

WHAT PEOPLE ARE SAYING...

"Karen Eubanks Jackson is a powerhouse. Her breast cancer journey is resilience, determination, and living your purpose in action. She reminds us all to turn our greatest challenge into an even bigger gift."
-**Tina Lifford**, actress, "**Queen Sugar**," author, *The Little Book of Big Lies: A Journey into Inner Fitness*

~

"Leadership. Vision. Compassion. Grace. Faithfulness. Endurance. These are the attributes of true leaders and agents of change and Karen E Jackson exemplifies each of these qualities and has for more than one third of her life. She is an admired hero who continues to lead Sisters Network in the fight against systemic injustice for all Black women. Karen began the national 501c-3 non-profit at a time when few people understood and not everyone supported. Yet she remained steadfast to support Sisters' legacy long before others even saw a need and with years of resistance, she persevered. Today, Sisters Network is part of the real conversation in establishing improved health care standards and practices to erasing disparities. What an amazing difference Karen Eubanks Jackson is making for the country."
-**Beverly Vote**, Publisher, **Breast Cancer Wellness Magazine**

~

"Stop The Silence" is tag line that truly has saved lives, specifically African American women. Before Sisters Network® Inc, African American women rarely thought about surviving breast cancer. To them, it was an automatic death sentence, even to African American women like my mother who had access. Karen's breast cancer journey is one of hope, faith and dedication, something she has been able to infuse in women throughout the network. She has devoted her life to building and spreading the message that African American women are not only survivors, but thrivers as well.

-**Lovell A. Jones,** Ph.D., F.H.D.R.
Professor Emeritus
University of Texas Distinguished Teaching Professor
University of Texas M.D. Anderson Cancer Center
University of Texas Graduate School of Biomedical Sciences

FOREWORD

BY LISA A. NEWMAN, MD

~

When Karen E. Jackson approached me to become the Chief National Medical Advisor for Sisters Network, I didn't hesitate at saying yes. As a surgical oncologist specializing in breast cancer, I know first-hand the devastating impact that a breast cancer diagnosis has on a woman. I also know that sisterhood is critical to patient well-being and cancer treatment recovery.

As a researcher, my primary focus has been on ethnicity-related variation in breast cancer risks and outcome with the goal of addressing current healthcare disparities in diagnosis, treatment and outcomes for women of color. While significant strides have been made in the medical community in regard to addressing breast cancer treatment disparities, there is much work that still needs to be done. African American women are still experiencing high breast cancer mortality rates and it is going to take grassroots advocacy and unity to address these deficiencies to improve the standard of care and outcomes.

And as an African American woman, I wanted to do anything I could to give my sisters hope on their journey.

Sisters Network provides a strong united front and a voice for women who often go unnoticed and unheard in the medical communities. Founder Karen Eubanks Jackson has proven that one person really can make a difference.

During her personal fight to survive breast cancer, she recognized a lack of "sisterhood" in traditional organizations. Despite a lack of vast resources or support, she worked tirelessly and never gave up. Her vision has come to full fruition with a national organization addressing the unique needs of African-American breast cancer survivors. Karen's primary motivation was to break through the silence and shame of breast cancer that immobilizes African American women, restricts their ability to receive support services, interferes with early detection, and ultimately affects their survival rates.

Sisters Network hosts the only annual national African-American Breast Cancer Conference and I was proud to serve as Honorary Chair for the tenth anniversary. Since its inception, the conference has attracted tens of thousands of African-American breast cancer survivors, their families, caretakers, and the general public, and general sessions are conducted by nationally recognized medical experts.

Because of Karen's advocacy, African-American women now have a real presence at leading breast cancer symposiums and increased participation in medical trials, which can eventually lead to improved treatments and better survival rates.

Recognizing the African American community's historical difficulty discussing cancer and other health concerns, Karen has served as a catalyst for change. Change that can mean the difference in life and death.

In the Company of My Sisters is a welcomed entry into the book marketplace and should be required reading for any sister who is about to embark on her own breast cancer journey.

Even though I am a doctor, I still find it heartbreaking when a woman presents with advanced stage breast cancer simply because she didn't know the signs or simply ignored the symptoms. Knowledge is power and Karen demonstrates both in her amazing life journey.

∾

Dr. Lisa A. Newman serves as Chief, Division of Breast Surgery, Director, Interdisciplinary Breast Program Weill Cornell Medicine/New York Presbyterian Hospital Network, New York, New York. Dr. Newman became interested in the disparities related to the breast cancer burden of African American women many years ago. This motivated her to pursue fellowship training in surgical oncology at M.D. Anderson Cancer Center to develop skills in conducting academic clinical research dedicated to understanding why African American women are more likely to develop advanced BC, and why AA have a younger age distribution for breast cancer. The study of breast cancer risk related to African ancestry has remained the main focus of her research. She is the founding medical director of an international breast cancer registry that features ongoing recruitment of multiethnic breast cancer patients from the United States (7 sites), Ghanaians/West Africans (2 sites) and Ethiopians/East Africans (2 sites). This position allows her to advance research related to breast cancer and genetic ancestry. In her current position as Director of the multidisciplinary breast oncology program for the Weill-Cornell/New York Presbyterian Hospital Network, Dr. Newman serves the Manhattan, Queens, and Brooklyn communities. The patient population, patient-centered outcome research expertise, and global research resources at Weill Cornell Medical College and New York Presbyterian Hospital allows her to optimize our initiatives for precision medicine and breast cancer disparities in a transdisciplinary fashion. Our international biorepository cohort has amassed over 3000 cases with tumor, blood and saliva samples for multi-omics, biomarker and germline risk studies. This unprecedented combination of patient diversity and cutting-

edge next generation technology has positioned us to lead the field in uncovering the distinctions in tumor biology that drive disparate outcomes of breast cancer across racial/ethnic strata. Interestingly, by virtue of our geographical catchment, we are also positioned to investigate questions related to environmental exposures to redefine how unique environmental factors may be drivers of distinct tumor biology. Together with the ICSBCS team, we are well-suited to carry out the proposed work of IGF-1 impact on tumor etiology.

INTRODUCTION

Dance as though no one is watching you
Love as though you have never been hurt
Sing as though no one can hear you
Live as though heaven is here on earth
- Anonymous

I remember the first time I heard the words: *You have breast cancer.*

It didn't really register with me then, which is crazy because before I knew, I *knew.* I knew something wasn't right with my body long before the doctors told me something was wrong.

When the doctor gave me that initial diagnosis, I didn't freak out. I just got real quiet. I was scared and didn't ask a lot of questions. I actually thought my diagnosis at the time meant that I only had five years to live. To this day I'm not even sure where I got that statistic from. But I was convinced that was my timeline. It all sounded fatal, and that's what I was initially processing. So I completely relate and understand how we as survivors hear and interpret information, no matter how much education and good sense we have.

That was in 1993 - a very bleak time to be a black breast cancer patient. The climate was hostile and lonely. Back then, I didn't know the first thing about the disease, except my aunt died in her 40's from it.

However, in true Karen Jackson mode, once the shock wore off, I went into a zone and absorbed information like I never had before about anything. Research became my friend, accompanying me everywhere I went. I attended support meetings and conferences and read any and everything I could. Talking about breast cancer consumed my life.

It didn't take me long to discover that finding information was difficult due to the limited amount of culturally-sensitive material. You learn quickly how to become your own best advocate and sometimes even your own best friend. And as I educated myself, the fire was fueled to educate others. In retrospect, my need to make a difference in the lives of black breast cancer survivors was my total focus.

This memoir is a culmination of my journey through breast cancer - from my personal experiences and observations as a survivor, to my life's path and commitment to increasing local and national attention, to the devastating impact that breast cancer has in the African-American community. And then, how just when I thought I'd beat the disease, it came back with a vengeance. Again and again and again.

This book has been 20 years in the making. But each time I began to write again, I became reinspired by the beauty and strength of the human spirit and I would want to change the course of the narrative.

I always carried the question: *How can you fully capture the essence of human life and how can you truly memorialize the loss of a loved one?*

It's been emotionally difficult losing so many members over

the years. At times, it has taken a tremendous toll on my well-being, but I chose to celebrate those women's lives through increased advocacy on their behalf. And in my efforts to advocate, the book kept getting sidelined.

Then my desire to tell this story became greater than my resistance to the obstacles that were in my path. My decision to shift my thinking from 'I don't have time to finish this story' to 'I need to *make* time to finish this story,' made the completion of this book of utmost importance.

It's funny because a great part of battling cancer required a shift in mindset. I'd mastered that, so the ability to take on unchartered territory was there from the beginning. I just had to shift that thinking and apply it to this book.

One thing I do know - for every woman who has lost her battle with cancer, there is a legacy that she leaves, and a spirit and light that continues to glow in the world. This book is in tribute to them. It's not only my story, my truth, but of the lessons learned from those who beat the disease – and those who sadly, didn't.

Sometimes when you learn of a breast cancer death, it's hard not to take it personally. You wonder if or when it may happen to you or a family member or friend. Once breast cancer touches your life, you are never quite the same, no matter how you attempt to move on. And believe it or not, this can be a good thing.

Today, because of advocacy, survivors are a powerful force in our society, thanks to their increasing numbers and visibility through media and community outreach. In addition, breast cancer support groups, and organizations such as the one I founded, Sisters Network Inc., offer an anchor to women diagnosed with this dreadful disease. The support from one another is invaluable. Members invest their own time and resources to share their personal journey with newly diagnosed members. There is no need for any woman to die from breast cancer uneducated about the disease, alone, or afraid.

We've accomplished so much, yet there is still so much to be done. We must continue to fight this disease with the strongest weapon in our arsenal: knowledge.

Women today have many roles - mother, daughter, wife, aunt, grandmother, neighbor, teacher, and last but certainly not least, SISTER. It's easy for us to lose ourselves in the quest to be all those things. But it's important to stay educated, enlightened, and inspired in the fight.

My life post-breast cancer has been richer and fuller. My life has a daily purpose, my relationships with others are enhanced and nurtured one day at a time, and I am truly grateful and blessed.

When you go to battle, you need a strong army. Sisters Network has been that for so many. If breast cancer had never affected me personally, I know that I would still be a supporter of the cause through financial support or by donating my time. It's a dreadful disease that no one should ignore or face alone.

I still don't have the answers to all the questions, but I do know that, together, we can accomplish so much. We are much stronger as a united force than we could ever be individually.

This book is written to give women the information and inspiration you need, answer questions you might have, and offer support you desire.

It's important to remember that you are not alone in your cancer battle. That's one of the lessons I hope you walk away having learned. Whether you're a survivor or a supporter, it is my hope that *In the Company of My Sisters* will help you navigate your breast cancer journey.

CHAPTER 1

IT ALL STARTS AT HOME

"All of my fundamental principles that were instilled in me in my home, from my childhood, are still with me. "
-Hakeem Olajuwon

I wasn't born with a silver spoon in my mouth. In fact, as a black girl growing up in Newark, New Jersey in the 1940s, my life was anything but easy. But values and a strong sense of self pride were so deeply instilled in me that I have always felt there was nothing I couldn't do.

Though my parents, John and Carliese Mason Eubanks struggled to raise their four children, they never wavered in their desire to give us a better life. My parents were hard-working, blue-collar workers. My father was a maintenance man at a telephone company, where he worked for fifty years, and my mother worked in an electrical factory and later went on to become a college musical director.

We lived in the "projects." But Baxter Terrance was home. And though the city-subsidized housing attracted low-income

1

working-class families, my parents always led us to believe poverty was a state of mind.

My brothers, Randall and Richard (and later my sister, Kimberly) and I never considered ourselves poor. As far as we were concerned, our parents simply worked hard with their eyes on a bigger prize.

"Daddy, why do you work so hard?" I remember once asking my father when he returned home from his job.

"Because there's something better for us on the other side," he told me, tussling my curly black hair.

That was my parent's motivation – that *something better.* They both dreamed of owning a home and moving to a nicer, integrated area.

When I was five, that dream became a reality.

My dad came home and announced that we were moving to Clinton Hill Section, into a modest, single-family, three-story house on Hillside Avenue in New Jersey.

I had never fully realized the economic challenges and social setbacks present for people of color because our daily experiences were rich. But I knew this move was major as my parents could barely contain their excitement.

After the move, and once we were settled in, I immediately noticed the difference in the greenery: the leaves and flowers in this neighborhood that we didn't have before. But the similarities were also noticeable. In Clinton Hill, the neighbors were friendly and kept a watchful eye on the children just like in Newark. Newark was experiencing "white flight" as more blacks were moving into the area, buying homes as a result of low-rate mortgages. So our new neighborhood was predominately white.

We were tested and enrolled in the Arts High School, a public school for performing arts and my parents encouraged our active participation in school and community social functions. And I ate it all up – participating in everything from cheerleading, choir, theater to sports.

An average student with no major discipline problems, I actually enjoyed going to school and learning new things. I've always been eager to learn and am very inquisitive. The schools my brothers and I attended were integrated, although some public establishments (restaurants, movie theatres, bathrooms, etc.) were still segregated.

Racism was rampant, though I don't have vivid memories of being treated differently in the classroom, or anywhere else for that matter, because I didn't recognize the signs.

My parents laid the foundation for our life success despite the tremendous financial and societal challenges they faced.

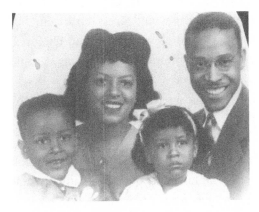

My mother, father, brother (Richard) and I.
-circa 1946. Mother wanted me to smile that day, I wished I had.

MOM AND DAD raised us with reasonable discipline and a strong sense of civic responsibility. Even as a young woman, I developed strong civic ethics and an appreciation of those values, which would be instrumental in my determination and vision to start a national organization with no outside funding and virtually no support outside of my immediate family.

I feel very fortunate to have been raised in a two-parent household. This is not to say that single-parent households cannot afford the same childhood experiences as two parents, but there are definite advantages to having both parents active in your life. Morals and values are reinforced collectively by two parents, instilling a strong sense of unity in the children through example.

As children, my brothers and I were made to feel that we could be anything we wanted to be. There were no limitations placed on us by our parents. That's something that resonates deep inside me to this day.

My childhood was full of family time, laughter, childhood play, and fond memories. Growing up the older daughter between two brothers (our baby sister, Kimberly, would join the family years later), I was a girly girl and a tomboy at the same time. My mother and I would dress up in our Sunday best - complete with hats and gloves and attend tea luncheons; but I also loved baseball, swimming, jump roping, and playing other sports with my brothers.

Of course, life was much simpler then and discipline was not questioned. When we misbehaved, a good ol' fashioned spanking would whip us back into shape. Mom and Dad were a disciplinary tag team. Mom was the stricter disciplinarian and Dad was the logical talker who would made us think about our actions and consequences. I could be sitting down with him playing a game of checkers and before I knew it, I just had a behavior counseling session. Discipline was a cornerstone in our structure and development.

While some people may have dreamed of having a more prosperous childhood, I'm actually thankful for my modest beginnings because a modest beginning can eventually turn into a remarkable finish.

CHAPTER 2

COMING OF AGE

"The maturing of a woman who has continued to grow is a beautiful thing to behold."
-Naomi Wolf

rom the time I was a young girl until I entered adulthood, or as they say now, adulting, I was captivated with glamour and fashion and aspired to be a fashionable lady of leisure. It was my mother's idea because, she worked extremely hard alongside my father and wanted a better educated, leisure life for me. That was why I always wanted more of the finer things in life. The fashion landscape was constantly changing and I did my best to keep up with it.

As I mentioned, I loved doing things outdoors. Up until about the age of twelve, I was considered a tomboy, following behind my big brother, Richard, playing baseball, riding bikes long distances, swimming...if there was something athletic to be done, I was game to do it. That's why I ended up with a four-inch scar on my right thigh, following my big brother.

Then one day, my mother simply said to me, "Karen, it's time to start becoming a young lady."

I believe her desire to mold me into a lady was what made me turn my interest to fashion. I always tried to make my mother proud, so I started following the modeling industry, reading designer books and magazines on clothes and homes.

By the time I was fourteen, I was all into my mother's makeover. In fact, she was so impressed with my commitment and dedication, she enrolled me into the top African American modeling school in New York City - the Althea DeVoe School of Modeling. Keep in mind we still lived in New Jersey. Paying for this training and traveling to New York City was very expensive but my family made yet another sacrifice and made it happen.

I soaked in all the modeling lessons, learning to walk, sit, talk and just look more sophisticated. I participated in fashion shows and beauty contests. During those days, in the fifties, having brown skin was not a plus, but I was not dismayed. I loved learning how to be poised and self-confident. Flipping through magazines while taking note of the latest beauty trends and fashions allowed me to visualize my life as a socialite and philanthropist living like the rich and famous, so I remained committed to soaking up everything I could.

Now, I've never been the type of person who idolized celebrities, and to this day I still don't get star struck. Though I respect their gifts and talent, at the end of the day, I feel they are no better than you or me. Celebrities face the same challenges as everyday people and that includes breast cancer. It doesn't discriminate. Notable celebrity breast cancer survivors include Ruby Dee, Naomi Sims, Hattie McDaniel, Diahann Carroll, Sheryl Crow, Olivia Newton John, Jaclyn Smith, Robin Roberts, Suzanne Summers, Roxie Roker, Cynthia Nixon, Alaina Reed-Hall, and model, Helen Williams.

Younger generations may not have the benefit of knowing

who Helen Williams was or what she came to stand for, but images of her were a defining point in my young life. Through my eyes, she was one of the most beautiful models of all time, black or white.

The copper-brown model was from Riverton, New Jersey, and went on to model for Dior in Paris. As I began to see more and more of her classic image in national advertisements, I started to look at my own reflection differently. I began to accept that my darker brown skin was beautiful. Prior to her emergence in the mainstream modeling arena, most of the models and women on television were white or light-skinned, and I was neither. So, she was a refreshing breath of air. She looked like me and that gave me hope.

Helen is regarded as the first black model to cross over into the mainstream market, and I was often told that I resembled her. She had a long, slender neck, polished hairstyles (the bouffant was popular at that time), and was the epitome of sophistication and poise.

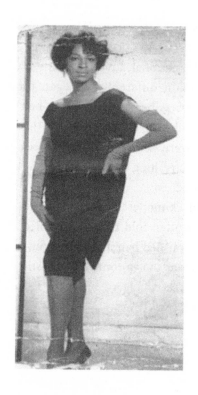

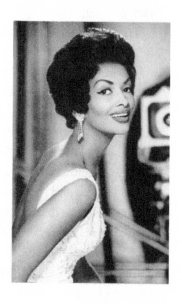

Me modeling a cape dress circa 1960
for a magazine ad at 17.
Paris model, Helen Williams.

EVEN THOUGH I enjoyed modeling and had some successes in the industry, I never intended it as a career. I was simply looking for a way to refine myself. So, when I graduated from high school, instead of doing like some of my fellow models and seeking full time work, I headed to Morgan State University in Baltimore, Maryland to gain an education and a husband.

In the early sixties, at seventeen, I was well-groomed, stylish and poised. But I went to college not knowing what to expect my first time in the south. I dressed stylishly, thinking that was how young women in college should dress.

I was wrong, not to mention out of touch with college fashion. My classmates were choosing comfort over beauty, and with my outfits, I was like a fish out of water. Even still, it did not change how I dressed.

Heading into college, my father let me know that he would pay for my education for two years because my brothers needed to get their degree more than I did. I understood and accepted what my father said. I attended Morgan for three years, then ended up marrying my college sweetheart, and having my daughter, Caleen.

We moved to Newark, New Jersey where I began working as a social worker and my husband was being groomed by the NBC Network to be an executive. Not long after the move, my husband was offered an amazing job in beautiful Los Angeles, California, so we were West Coast bound.

I was excited to move in the early seventies and proud to be the wife of an executive. My plan was to be a stay-at-home wife and helpmate.

You know what they say about the best-laid plans...

My marriage ended about two years after moving to California. I concentrated on raising my beautiful daughter and starting a new life for me.

Being a young mother in Los Angeles was exciting, especially coming from New Jersey. Since I'd gotten married straight out of college, this was my first time living on my own. That may have been scary for many women, but I embraced the change and challenge even though my parents thought it was best I return back home to New Jersey.

I found my entrepreneurial spirit, used my fashion interests, got training, and ended up working several different jobs in the makeup industry.

While still in Los Angeles, I met my second husband a few years later and we were married for about fifteen years. The size of our family increased because he had six children who lived with us off and on. He was a general contractor so we moved around, which gave us the opportunity to live in different cities. That was interesting because the cities were all so different, in good and bad ways.

I used my talents in design to help in building his business. His work would eventually take us back to California and we ended up divorced shortly after. But I enjoyed being single again. Though I was a single mother, I decided to go to cosmetology school, where I got my license and then opened a hair weaving business in Beverly Hills.

For me, the future looked bright.

CHAPTER 3

DON'T ASK, DON'T TELL

"There are some secrets that we think we're keeping, but those secrets are actually keeping us."
-Frank Warren

I've come to realize that our vision for our lives may not be what we intended, but instead, what God intended. Faith and the church played a large part in my upbringing in my early years. As a family, we attended church together regularly, and my grandmother not only played the organ but led the choir. Attendance and participation in church was a substantial part of our upbringing. The church is where our morals, values, and the importance of respecting our elders were reinforced.

There have always been certain topics of conversation that are taboo in the black church and the black community, in general, and illness ranks high on that list. In my experience, black people are still a very private group when it comes to sharing personal struggles. I remember being asked to leave the room when "grown folks were talking,"; it wasn't appropriate to have adult conversations in the presence of children.

One of my mother's sisters died of breast cancer in her late forties. All of my aunts were special to me, but this particular aunt was my favorite when I was a little girl. I loved everything about my Aunt Cleo: she made me laugh, was very outspoken, and overall was just a fun woman to be with. She left behind one son and one daughter when she passed. I didn't know much about her illness except that she was hospitalized and seemed to die suddenly. There just wasn't much discussion about her illness or death; we were just supposed to accept it and silently move on.

Later, when I received my first diagnosis, I asked my mother about Aunt Cleo's death.

"I need to know our family history," I told my mother one day.

"For what?" she replied.

"Because I need to know. Isn't breast cancer why Aunt Cleo died? I've never had details and really would like to know."

"I don't want to talk about that, Sweetheart," she replied. "But I will tell you your grandfather's sister aunt Emma had a double mastectomy and she died, too."

I was dumbfounded. All these years and no one in my family had ever mentioned that. But then I found out that no one knew until her death as she never shared her diagnosis. It wasn't until she was getting prepped for the funeral that most of the family learned she had underwent a double mastectomy. Again, it was something no one talked about. My great-aunt died in silence and alone with no one to share her challenges.

That lack of knowledge made both deaths even more traumatic for those of us who were left behind.

Breast cancer, or even the word breasts, just wasn't something you talked about openly. But we were very much aware of heart disease and diabetes. Several family members suffered from those issues and everyone spoke freely about their struggles.

But we never talked about cancer. Back in those days, cancer was like a black cloud that never went away. When a woman was diagnosed with breast cancer, it was always anticipated that she would have a long, drawn-out, and painful death.

With such a strong history of breast cancer affecting the women in my family, I went off into the world as a young woman with a little voice always gnawing in the back of my mind.

It would whisper to me, *"Be diligent in your health."*

"Take good care of your body."

"Always seek medical attention when something doesn't feel quite right."

That inner voice would save my life.

CHAPTER 4

A WOMAN'S INTUITION

"Follow your instincts. That's where true wisdom manifests itself."
-Oprah Winfrey

*W*omen are very intuitive creatures. Our intuition is our inner guidance tool. A woman's ability to tap into her higher wisdom gives her the ability to look inward to her understanding of the world that encompasses her. I credit my intuition with saving my life through early-stage breast cancer detection.

Breast cancer touches so many lives on so many levels. It is the most common cancer among American women and the number-two killer of women in the U.S.

Breast cancer occurs when cells in the tissues of the breast become abnormal and divide without order or control. These malignant cells form too much tissue and become a tumor that can grow into nearby tissue or cells. The tumor can also break away, and enter the bloodstream or lymphatic system, which has the potential to affect other organs.

In 2020 (the latest figures at the time this book was written), an estimated 276,480 new cases of invasive breast cancer are expected to be diagnosed in women in the U.S., along with 48,530 new cases of non-invasive breast cancer.

Some other statistics worth noting:

- About 1 in 8 U.S. women (about 12%) will develop invasive breast cancer over the course of her lifetime.
- About 42,170 women in the U.S. are expected to die in 2020 from breast cancer. Death rates have been steady in women under 50 since 2007 but have continued to drop in women over 50. The overall death rate from breast cancer decreased by 1.3% per year from 2013 to 2017. These decreases are thought to be the result of treatment advances and earlier detection through screening.
- In women under 45, breast cancer is more common in black women than white women. Overall, black women are more likely to die of breast cancer.
- For women in the U.S., breast cancer death rates are higher than those for any other cancer, with the exception of lung cancer.
- As of January 2020, there are more than 3.5 million women with a history of breast cancer in the U.S. This includes women currently being treated and women who have finished treatment.
- Besides skin cancer, breast cancer is the most commonly diagnosed cancer among American women. In 2020, it's estimated that about 30% of newly diagnosed cancers in women will be breast cancer.
- Breast cancer incidence rates in the U.S. began decreasing in the year 2000, after increasing for the previous two decades. They dropped by 7% from

2002 to 2003 alone. One theory is that this decrease was partially due to the reduced use of hormone replacement therapy (HRT) by women after the results of a large study called the Women's Health Initiative were published in 2002. These results suggested a connection between HRT and increased breast cancer risk. In recent years, incidence rates have increased slightly by 0.3% per year.

- A woman's risk of breast cancer nearly doubles if she has a first-degree relative (mother, sister, daughter) who has been diagnosed with breast cancer. Less than 15% of women who get breast cancer have a family member diagnosed with it.

- About 5-10% of breast cancers can be linked to known gene mutations inherited from one's mother or father. Mutations in the *BRCA1* and *BRCA2* genes are the most common. On average, women with a *BRCA1* mutation have up to a 72% lifetime risk of developing breast cancer. For women with a *BRCA2* mutation, the risk is 69%. Breast cancer that is positive for the *BRCA1* or *BRCA2* mutations tends to develop more often in younger women. An increased ovarian cancer risk is also associated with these genetic mutations. In men, *BRCA2* mutations are associated with a lifetime breast cancer risk of about 6.8%; *BRCA1* mutations are a less frequent cause of breast cancer in men.

- About 85% of breast cancers occur in women who have no family history of breast cancer. These occur due to genetic mutations that happen as a result of the aging process and life in general, rather than inherited mutations.

- The most significant risk factors for breast cancer are sex (being a woman) and age (growing older).

American Cancer Society

No single trigger or cause has been identified for breast cancer, but there are certain risk factors that may increase a woman's chance of developing it. Some of those factors include:

- **Age** - it's more common in women over fifty.
- **Family history** - if a woman's mother or sister had the disease before menopause, this is occasionally associated with one of two genes linked to breast cancer. Family history of ovarian cancer is another factor.
- **Age of pregnancy** - women who haven't had children or who were over the age of thirty when their first child was born.
- **Age of menstruation** - starting periods at a young age (under twelve years old).
- **Entering menopause** later (over age fifty-five).
- **Smoking** - Recent research suggests that women who start smoking regularly within five years of the onset of their menstrual periods are seventy percent more likely to develop breast cancer before the age of fifty than non-smokers.
- **Having dense breast tissue.**
- **Radiation treatment** to the chest, especially before thirty years of age.
- **Excessive alcohol** consumption.
- **Hormone replacement therapy** (HRT: estrogen plus progesterone) increases the risk of breast cancer slightly after five years of therapy.
- **Oral contraceptives** increase risks slightly if used over many years.

- **Obesity** with excess caloric and fat intake.

HAVING HAD SUCH a strong family history of breast cancer, I knew the odds were most likely not in my favor. I knew there was a strong chance that I would develop breast cancer, but I strongly believe that we are never given more than we can handle. The key to overcoming any obstacle is to prepare ahead of time to beat it.

My time came in 1993.

I was living in the beautiful city of Los Angeles with my husband, Kyle, running a successful hair weaving business, and loving life. Kyle was a successful actor who was actively working, and things were going very well for us. My only child, Caleen, was engaged, and living and working as a successful public relations practitioner in Houston, TX. It was a really great point in all of our lives. And then, cancer decided to rear its ugly head.

I was an athletically active person who took great care of my appearance and health and due to my strong family history of breast cancer, I'd begun doing routine self-breast exams at a rather early age.

One morning while getting dressed, I felt a new and suspicious lump on the right side of my breast between the areola and underarm in what is referred to as quadrant four.

I started having mammograms at the age of thirty-five because I was fortunate enough to have health coverage that supported this and, once again, based on my family history, I was more aware of the need to be proactive in early detection. I believed in going to the doctor regularly and relying on medical experts.

Growing up, going to the doctor was never an unpleasant experience for me. I would accompany my parents to the doctor and we never hesitated to seek medical attention, so I kept that mentality into adulthood.

After a couple of years of getting mammograms, I felt as though there was something wrong. I'd had several mammograms and nothing ever showed up. Nothing was hurting, but in my research, I'd learned that breast cancer doesn't hurt, though I was feeling sensations.

So, when I found the lump, I knew that I needed to have a mammogram to confirm. What I didn't know was that an ultrasound would be the second step. But it was I, listening to my body, who knew that a second step was needed.

And so, though he didn't want to, my doctor recommended the ultrasound. He felt that I was being overly concerned, but he finally recommended it because I had been with him for several years. My mammogram had shown that everything was good, but I knew it wasn't. My inner spirit just told me it wasn't. So, I finally I got up enough courage to demand that he give me the next appointment that was available for the ultrasound.

Lo and behold, I took the ultrasound and I had a 3.5 centimeter cancer, but it wasn't a calcification, a common process where small spots of calcium deposit themselves in breast tissue. These deposits can be the result of aging or other breast conditions such as fibroadenoma or cysts and are often detected on mammograms.

Despite having prior mammograms in that region of my breast, that particular area continued to weigh on my spirit. It turned out to be a palatable mast, which is fleshy tissue. So, there was no way to feel extra flesh. It was just there.

I wasn't comfortable with the calcification diagnosis and was so glad that I demanded the ultrasound to determine exactly what it was. When you have concerns about something, you should always follow your instincts. When you are fully in tune with your body, you can detect when something is out of sync.

The lump in question turned out to be a palpable mass with a diameter of 3.5 cm.

After the ultrasound finding, a biopsy was scheduled that would remove tissue or fluid from my breast to be looked at under a microscope for further testing.

There are different kinds of biopsies: fine needle aspiration, core biopsy, or open biopsy. In 1993, biopsies took several days to come back with a result. Many survivors and their loved ones agree that waiting for test results causes anxiety, stress, and even insomnia. Thankfully, I was able to get results within a few hours, but unfortunately, it was confirmed that the mass was malignant.

At that moment, I was simply dumbfounded and numb. I wasn't completely caught off guard because I already had my suspicions about the lump. That particular area had a tingling and I was experiencing a strange sensation. My intuition led me to believe that it might be cancer and although I anticipated the news, I wasn't prepared to accept it. I was still caught completely off guard.

I never just sat and cried during my diagnosis, treatment, or recovery phase. It's not that I view crying as a sign of weakness; it's just that I am generally a person who does not cry a lot. My husband and daughter can attest to this. Tears may have welled up, but they never fell. You can't shed tears over what you haven't accepted, and I was strongly in denial. Plus, I was too busy planning on how I was going to treat the cancer rather than spend that time crying, which wasn't going to solve anything.

∽

"OUR FIRST REACTION WAS FEAR. You're not ever ready to hear 'you have cancer'. I had a long family history of cancer, including my mom, aunts, and uncles, and I was scared to death. Karen was never angry,

and she never cried. She was deeply in denial. She didn't realize the depth of her illness until halfway through her chemo treatments. It was heartbreaking for me to watch her go through chemo, especially when it started to physically wear her down."

-Kyle Jackson, husband of 34 years

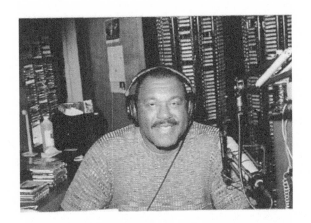

CHAPTER 5

LIFTING THE FOG

"Healing is the result of clear thinking."
-Ernest Holmes

Since I wasn't able to clearly think, I wasn't capable of making good decisions about my health or treatment at the time. This was where my husband and daughter readily stepped in and I easily let them lead. I could function in any other way but not in this area. I also became deeply withdrawn.

I was unable to think how and what my next steps should be. I was able to handle my hair business, home, etc., but made no decisions on my care.

Fortunately, my family made good decisions on my behalf. Kyle, my husband, took me to all my treatments and we discussed everything together.

I had a choice of a mastectomy or lumpectomy and opted for a lumpectomy, a new option offered during this time that was less invasive. It would remove the cancerous tissue and a small amount of normal tissue around the lump. When considering surgical choices, each woman needs to think about her type of cancer, her physician's recommendations, family history, the risk of recurrence, and, of course, any anticipated body image concerns.

After the lumpectomy, I experienced moderate pain and was sent home the next day with two Jackson-Pratt (JP) drainage tubes near my rib cage. A Jackson-Pratt drain is a device used to pull excess fluid from the body by constant suction.

Twelve lymph nodes were removed for testing, but none tested positive for cancer. This was prior to the development of the sentinel node biopsy procedure, which would have involved removing only one node, testing it, and lessening my likelihood of later developing lymphedema.

Lymphedema, also known as lymphatic obstruction, is a painful condition of localized fluid retention and tissue swelling caused by a compromised lymphatic system. It usually presents itself as an aching or feeling of fullness in the arm or breast. Early treatment is very important to decrease swelling. Anytime lymph nodes are removed, the patient is at risk of developing this condition.

Telling my mother that I had breast cancer was extremely difficult because she started relating my diagnosis to the death of my aunts, Cleo and Emma, but she handled it very well. She was there for me and I never saw her break down or cry.

When it came time to have my surgery, she showed up at the hospital. My father had just died so she was having a hard time emotionally. I was preparing to go into surgery and she said, "I can't do this."

I was stunned.

"I can't handle my child being operated on," she said. "I'm just going to go home."

I have to admit, I was disappointed and hurt, especially because my mother and I were so close. But looking back, I understand. Like most in my family, it wasn't something that she wasn't comfortable talking about, let alone witnessing. Add to that the extreme grief she was still processing from my father's death and she simply wasn't herself.

There were ten days between my surgery and Caleen's wedding and I was her event planner for her wedding. My mind was not focused on my breast cancer or surgery, but rather being well enough to fulfill the position of event planner and mother of the bride. Everything went fairly well post-surgery as far as my physical recovery was concerned. Luckily, I have a high pain threshold.

"MOM'S DIAGNOSIS really caught me off guard. In fact, I was speechless. Simply put, Mom was amazing through it all. She was so unselfish and continued to put me first. I practically begged her to allow me to postpone my upcoming wedding but she wasn't having it. She was determined not to let cancer bring her down or stop the show."

-Caleen Burton-Allen, daughter

I WAS DETERMINED that my daughter was going to have a perfect wedding and so I went over every detail several times. Though it had only been ten days since my surgery, I continued doing all that it took to make sure all things regarding the wedding, including the reception for the wedding party, went off without any problems.

I remained in bed during the wedding rehearsals, but I rose to the occasion when it was show time. In fact, hardly anyone knew about my diagnosis, with the exception of a few bridal attendants, but the general wedding attendees were unaware.

The day of the wedding, I was in the hotel room getting dressed. I was feeling tired but happy about my daughter's day. I had my outfit on, a designer suit that I'd especially picked out for this occasion. And then, I passed the full-length mirror in the hotel room. I stood there, taking in my appearance, admiring the suit I'd meticulously chosen.

And being saddened at the sight of the draining tubes coming out of the side of my breast.

I tried to work with the tubes, adjusting and readjusting to hide them. Since we were at the hotel already and I didn't have a substitute outfit. I tucked and re-tucked, shifted the tubes from side to side and up and down. To no avail. They were still obvious under my outfit.

I stood in front of the mirror that day, looking at the woman I had become. I was battling breast cancer - determined to beat it - and it was about to mess up my daughter's special day.

Something came over me and I grabbed the tube and started pulling. I ignored the voice inside me saying, 'What are you doing?' I silenced the internal voice screaming, 'Put it back in!' And I just kept pulling.

The tube was at least a yard long. I stood in the hotel room with it clutched tightly in my hand and felt momentarily victorious. And then my eyes made their way back to the mirror and I gasped at the hole in my body.

I stared at myself for a few minutes, then inhaled, set the tube on the counter, grabbed some padding to cover the hole and catch the fluid as it continued to drain, put my suit back on and made my way downstairs to watch my baby girl.

Of course, I don't advise anyone doing anything like that. But that was my 'take charge' moment. (It's a blessing the pad nor fluid never showed through my clothes.) It was a crazy move and could've been dangerous, but even now if I had to do it over again, I would do the exact same thing.

People may not understand why I pulled my tubes out, but I absolutely did not want to take anything away from Caleen's special day or cause unnecessary attention to myself. Although she wanted to call the wedding off, I demanded that the wedding go on and I refused to let my breast cancer interrupt her wedding day or our lives.

After the wedding, my close friends told me that I "appeared larger than the room," and my daughter's friends told me that Caleen had been hysterical with worry about me, though she kept it from me.

I guess we both were trying to protect each other.

I confided in my sister and sister-in-law after the surgery, but there was not much they could do since they lived out of town.

Ultimately, it was my daughter who took control of the situation. After the wedding, she remained in Texas and I was still in California, but she immediately went into action. Caleen channeled all of her journalism research skills and found the UCLA Cancer Center in California for me. I was so grateful for that. Again, I wasn't thinking clearly, and neither was my husband. In fact, I wasn't even thinking about moving. I knew that I had to get to the hospital for the surgery, but I didn't really think beyond that. And I definitely didn't know I would have to go through a cancer treatment center.

I eventually gave up my hair care business due to concerns I had about the loss of strength in my right hand from the treatment and removal of my lymph nodes. I obviously needed to use my hands for my job so I knew it was time to let the business go. I didn't get too depressed about not working, but I started giving some serious thought to what else I was going to do with the rest of my life.

When I was first diagnosed, I was told that because of my general overall health and stage II cancer diagnosis (invasive ductal carcinoma) chemotherapy and radiation could be done together and would be well tolerated.

The chemo regimen I had would cause my hair to thin but not completely fall out. Hair follicles are weakened by chemotherapy and causes your hair to fall out much more quickly than it would normally. It typically occurs anywhere between days seven and twenty-one after the first chemotherapy dosing. I know that most cancer patients, especially young women, find the hair loss traumatic and sometimes devastating, but I was not overly concerned with it.

When I found out it would grow back, that was one less worry off my plate. Plus, having worked in the hair business I knew the hottest tricks-of-the-trade when it came to weaves, wigs, and extensions.

I received the chemotherapy via vascular access through an arm vein, since the chest catheter, or port, also known as the Port-A-Cath, was not an option at that time. In a vascular access procedure, a special catheter is inserted inside a major vein (generally in one of the large veins in the neck or in the arm) extending into the large central vein near the heart.

I was already sleeping a lot after my surgery, but then almost immediately after the first treatment, I felt sick and even more tired during adjuvant therapy. My chemo treatment was administered at the University of California Los Angeles Jonsson Cancer Center, internationally renowned for innovative cancer research and the best in cancer diagnosis, treatment, and prevention in Los Angeles and throughout Southern California. I received my chemotherapy treatment over six months.

My husband would drive me to the center and stay with me the entire time. Leaving, I was so exhausted I would never make it home without falling asleep in the car.

Initially, the drip cycle was given over a two-hour period, but that proved to be too strong of a dosage, so it had to be adjusted.

It is common practice for the second and subsequent chemotherapies to require adjustment once your oncologist gauges how you react to the initial dosing. Many patients develop a condition called neutropenia when treated for cancer with chemotherapy drugs. The term neutropenia describes the situation where the number of neutrophils in the blood is too low. Neutrophils are very important in defending the body against bacterial infections, and, therefore, a patient with too few neutrophils is more susceptible to bacterial infections. Neutropenia almost always requires a hospital stay and this can be a distressing time if the patient doesn't know what to expect.

By my third chemo, I tried to decline treatment. I was mentally, emotionally, and physically drained. Once I mentally allowed myself to believe that the chemo medications were beneficial to me, and were killing the cancer, my body did not get as sick. It was a mind over matter situation.

There are so many side effects from chemotherapy and each person will respond differently. Some side effects that I vividly recall include dry mouth with a metallic taste and instant hot flashes. Survivors like to refer to these hot flashes as "power surges."

I received radiation at the same time as chemo and it was extremely taxing on me. Nowadays, chemo and radiation are usually given separately with time in between to allow the body to heal.

Fortunately, we had good insurance so it didn't bankrupt us, but it could have. The procedures were so expensive, not to mention time-consuming. I was going every day for six weeks for the radiation, then weekly for the chemotherapy. Radiation takes your energy and the chemotherapy makes you sick. So, the combination made for a rough six months.

There were times when I felt like I wasn't going to survive because of the physical pain and the emotional turmoil of my family history. But I made it. I was grateful for my family support, for having insurance and for ongoing healing. Yet and still, I felt like something was missing. I needed to talk to other women who looked like me who were going through this journey. I needed sisterhood.

CHAPTER 6

IN SEARCH OF SISTER

"Don't walk in front of me; I may not follow.
Don't walk behind me; I may not lead.
Just walk beside me and be my friend."
- Albert Camus

uring my visits to the cancer center, I didn't interact or even see many black patients during chemotherapy. I developed a strong yearning to reach out and talk to someone who could fully understand what I was going through and how I was feeling. It wasn't that I couldn't talk to my family and friends, but there was only so much they could understand or absorb.

From the moment I'd been diagnosed with breast cancer, I'd never been ashamed. I just immediately thought, how long will I live with breast cancer?

I shared my story every chance I got. When I went to church or to another social event or when someone asked, 'how are you doing?' I just opened up.

I wanted to talk about it and no one - not even the family I loved dearly - could stop me.

I had a story to tell and I was ready to tell it.

I did manage to meet new people and instantly bonded with other patients. One person in particular was a woman who was bringing her mother in for colon cancer treatments and she would sit with her mom during her chemo. The daughter and I were around the same age and her mom was my mother's age. I enjoyed our talks and actually looked forward to seeing them when I had chemo.

Upon completion of treatment, we lost touch with one another and I realized that I needed that ongoing support to help me get through this emotionally.

One of my major observations through participation with other cancer-related support groups was that the educational focus centered on white patients and the support tended to end when the treatment ended. During sessions, I sat and talked, and shared stories, but there wasn't a long-term connection or new relationships forged.

I was so happy to complete my chemo and radiation treatments and celebrated with friends and family feeling a huge sense of relief and accomplishment.

Survivors celebrated this milestone with gatherings at home, restaurants, or even at the treatment center with balloons and refreshments. Completing a phase of treatment was a tremendous milestone. From day one, I just wanted it to be done. But where did I go from here?

With that mindset, I packed up and moved to Houston to be with my only child. Kyle was not initially on board. He didn't think it was a good idea. But thankfully, he quickly realized that the two of us needed to do this together. He was a working actor so he was able to move.

Being close to Caleen and fully living life (what I thought I had left of it) was the most important thing to me. But there was still that inner voice telling me to do something for my "sisters" on a grand scale. The lack of unified leadership to address breast cancer disparities was a calling that I could not ignore.

PRIOR TO RELOCATING to Houston in 1994, I was already entertaining the thought of starting a national organization to provide support for African American breast cancer survivors. Almost immediately after my own diagnosis, I actively started seeking out other women who looked like me for camaraderie and conversation regarding what they knew about breast cancer. I also had a strong desire to seek out other survivors to ask questions, find out if they were interested in a breast cancer organization, and gain intimate knowledge of their diagnosis and treatment.

It was comforting to talk to someone who was already finished or somebody who was ahead of you, even though we may not be taking the same chemo. I felt a need to compare myself to other survivors so I could measure how I was really doing. There were questions that only a person who had gone through breast cancer could answer, like how did the radiation feel? Was I healing normally? Did my scar appear different? Would my body ever fully recover? Reading a book or pamphlet about breast cancer was not enough for me.

"You've been getting ready to take on the system from the start," my best friend, Yvonne, told me one day.

She was right. I was angry with what I saw as injustices, the education being universal, the atmosphere, the approach of different associations, chemo wasn't regulated properly...there was a difference in so much when it came to treating breast cancer. Some people had to wait, go through the system, etc. in order to have their surgeries. I realized that in order for people to know what they were getting they had to know their choices.

So I immediately went to work on behalf of the cause. Breast cancer patients needed to talk to other women who had the disease in a support group setting. Where you lack understanding, search for it until you get it. You can't make wise choices if you are not fully informed.

For me specifically, it was a deep-down desire for human interaction with other women battling breast cancer. I wanted to encourage women to be open about their survivor status. The more united and open, the more women we could reach and free them from their silence.

I was relieved that the chains of silence were slowly being broken, but not everyone was supportive of my outspokenness. My own mother struggled to understand why I wanted to tell anybody about my personal cancer battle. She disagreed with me for a few years for sharing my story publicly, which goes back to the long-held belief in the black community that you should deal with certain illnesses privately. I can't stress it enough: when it comes to breast cancer, silence is never golden.

My daughter and husband liked to tease that I practically "accosted" any women of color and talked to her at great lengths about breast cancer. If you were in line behind me at the supermarket or post office, more likely than not, you were going to have a breast cancer discussion aimed at you.

My vision was for black women to be more engaged in breast cancer awareness as community advocates. In the start-up stage, my vision was larger than anything else. I didn't have vast resources, but I was determined to fulfill my dream. Establishing a network of sisterhood support became my newfound purpose in life.

So, I started studying and reading up and educating myself, going to conferences, going to support groups. I was surprised that I couldn't pick up the phone and call an 800 number and find an African American national organization. That was shocking to me. I thought that information would be easy to find; I just assumed it would be. And when I found out not only was there not a telephone number, but there was no organization at all, my mind went into overdrive.

I looked at everything that was going on in the breast cancer arena and how we were perceived as black women - that we didn't care about our health, that we didn't follow up on our doctor's visits. Everything I read was about what we didn't do, never mind what the cancer was doing to us. I found that very offensive because having had family support, having had the money and insurance to get proper treatment, I still would have fallen through the cracks early on if my daughter hadn't researched to find the cancer center. The surgeon didn't suggest a cancer center or provide guidance on what to do afterward. He simply removed the tumor and I never saw him again. So I knew that my lack of knowledge could have been detrimental and made my journey a whole lot worse because I just didn't know.

So that propelled me into thinking that if I, an educated person, could lose my life just because I didn't know something, imagine the millions of women who were out there. I started trying to think of what it would take to educate women like me.

One of the most pressing things I discovered was that, at that time, the health professionals didn't know or have a name for triple negative breast cancer, which is the most serious breast cancer because it gets to the women at an earlier age and it's more aggressive. So any woman, at that time, who was getting triple negatives (which I didn't get) could have a serious condition.

The more I learned, the more I wanted to share. I felt the need to share my story with people who understood what I was going through. Again, it wasn't that my friends and family weren't there, but if a woman hasn't had breast cancer, she really can't relate to what you have to go through. I believe a woman has to walk the walk and talk to talk in order to really truly know what another woman is going through. And no one goes through it the same way. Two women can have the same breast cancer, stage two or one or whatever. But how a woman feels about it and how she feels about her body makes a difference.

There was so much I'd learned. And I wanted to share it all.

CHAPTER 7

EDUCATION IS KEY

"A lack of knowledge creates fear. Seeking knowledge creates courage."
                                                    -Candice Swanepoel

This much I know: a lack of knowledge can prove detrimental in the battle against breast cancer.

That's why educating women has been my passion for years and I've found some basic areas where we need educating the most.

The different types of cancer

First of all, many people don't know that there are different types of cancers. When you say breast cancer, everybody thinks it's the same thing but it's not. My knowledge of breast cancer was very limited in the beginning. Even though I knew I had a family history, there was still so much I didn't know.

One of the first things I discovered was that there are many types of breast cancer, and many different ways to describe each illness.

The type of breast cancer a woman has been diagnosed with is determined by the specific cells in the breast that are affected. Most breast cancers are *carcinomas*, which are tumors that start in the epithelial cells that line organs and tissues throughout the body. When carcinomas form in the breast, they are usually a more specific type called *adenocarcinoma*, which starts in cells in the ducts (the milk ducts) or the lobules (milk-producing glands).

In situ vs. invasive breast cancers

The type of breast cancer can also refer to whether the cancer has spread or not. Situ breast cancer (ductal carcinoma in situ or DCIS) is a cancer that starts in a milk duct and has not grown into the rest of the breast tissue. The term *invasive (or infiltrating) breast cancer* is used to describe any type of breast cancer that has spread (invaded) into the surrounding breast tissue.

Ductal carcinoma in situ (DCIS)

Ductal carcinoma in situ (DCIS; also known as *intraductal carcinoma*) is a non-invasive or pre-invasive breast cancer.

Some invasive breast cancers have special features or develop in different ways that affect their treatment and outlook. These cancers are less common but can be more serious than other types of breast cancer.

Invasive breast cancer (ILC or IDC)

Invasive (or infiltrating) breast cancer means the cancer has spread into surrounding breast tissue. The most common types are *invasive ductal carcinoma* and *invasive lobular carcinoma*. Invasive ductal carcinoma makes up about 70-80% of all breast cancers.

Triple-negative breast cancer

Triple-negative breast cancer is an aggressive type of invasive breast cancer that accounts for about 15% of all breast cancers. It is a difficult cancer to treat.

Inflammatory breast cancer

Inflammatory breast cancer is an uncommon type of invasive cancer. It accounts for about 1% to 5% of all breast cancers.

There are some less common types of breast cancer, that

affect various cells in the breast. These cancers are much less common, and sometimes need different types of treatment.

PAGET DISEASE of the breast

Paget disease of the breast starts in the breast ducts and spreads to the skin of the nipple and then to the areola (the dark circle around the nipple). It is rare, accounting for only about 1-3% of all cases of breast cancer.

Angiosarcoma

Sarcomas of the breast are rare making up less than 1% of all breast cancers. Angiosarcoma starts in cells that line blood vessels or lymph vessels. It can involve the breast tissue or the skin of the breast. Some may be related to prior radiation therapy in that area.

Phyllodes tumor

Phyllodes tumors are rare breast tumors. They develop in the connective tissue (stroma) of the breast, in contrast to carcinomas, which develop in the ducts or lobules. Most are benign, but there are others that are malignant (cancer).

BY NO MEANS am I a doctor, so it's imperative that you allow your doctor to give you an official diagnosis. (You'd be stunned at the number of people who try to self-diagnose.) I just believe that when you enter your doctor's office, you should be armed with an arsenal of information.

One of the biggest things I discovered in my research is that self-advocacy could help save our lives. The problem was that black women especially, didn't even know what questions to ask. We were lacking so much, we didn't know, what we didn't know. At the time, I thought I only had five years to live (remember that self-imposed timeline I'd given myself), so I was dedicated during those first five years to make a difference.

My desire to educate others gave me more fuel to keep me going because I was intent on delivering better answers than what women currently had access to.

I was meeting women from across the country who had insurance and had everything in play, yet they're not here today because they selected the wrong hospital or the wrong doctor or they went into a depression so bad that they didn't even want to eat or do anything. Fear immobilizes some women, causing them not to make a decision or take action. While education won't always change that, knowledge is still power.

Everyone's journey is unique and what you bring to the table of breast cancer will help determine your survival chances. It really does matter. And if you have knowledge, you have some power.

I've seen it over and over again with the members of Sisters Network, Inc., particularly in Florida. One of our members there was told to make arrangements for her passing because there was nothing else anyone could do for her.

She did research herself and found her way to MD Anderson Cancer Center in Houston. Twenty years later, she's still here.

If she had listened to her local physician who, for whatever reason, didn't know about the new techniques or the newest research, or the type of cancer that she was battling, or even his own implicit biases...if she'd accepted his dismal diagnosis, she wouldn't be here.

That is a prime example of why it's imperative to be your own self-advocate (I'll talk more about that later).

She and I worked together to make sure she got at least that first, second and third opinion. If MD Anderson had told her there wasn't anything they could do, then I would have had her go to another hospital. Hospitals and doctors don't all agree. I discovered that by going to medical conferences.

And that's also why you have to have enough knowledge

about the cancer itself, your own body, and what you're willing to do.

I've also discovered that health professionals are often so focused on treating your body that they don't include treating your mind. If you mentally fight against the chemo when you're taking it, it doesn't work as well. You have to tell yourself, 'this is going to save my life. I'm submitting myself to this and I'm going to live.' This is one situation where I can attest that attitude is everything.

And as scary as this all can be, you have to shake off the fear. Fear keeps people from even going to get the mammogram and learning that they have breast cancer.

I met one such woman at a gala in Houston. She was an accountant with her own business. She was in her forties and the epitome of professionalism.

"Hello, Mrs. Jackson, I know this is highly unusual, but I respect your work with breast cancer a lot. Do you have a minute to step in the restroom so I can show you something?" she asked.

I'd had this type of thing happen before, so I wasn't taken aback. I followed her into the bathroom, and I saw the fear in her eyes as she lifted her blouse to reveal a gauze covering her breast.

"I think something is wrong," she said, as she gently lifted the bandage.

I looked on in shock. Something was definitely wrong. She had cancer growing out of her body - literally. I was well-educated by that point, but I had never seen an open wound like that. It looked like an ulcer on her breast. It was open, fluid was oozing out, and it had an odor.

"I know something is wrong," she said, fighting back tears. "I look at this every day."

"Have you been to a doctor?" I asked, already knowing the answer.

"No. I'm scared," she replied.

After talking with her some more, I discovered she was an educated woman in denial. She could look in the mirror, see the wound, even smell it and know something was wrong, but she was scared of what the doctors would say.

I ended up going with her to the doctor. I'm glad I did. She went to a doctor in her healthcare plan and I could instantly tell he was not giving her the best advice. I knew that the new protocol was to have the chemo to shrink the cancer and then remove it by surgery. This doctor didn't know that, or just didn't offer that as an option.

So, we left to find someone who was going to give her the best way of treating her cancer.

Her fear was palpable. I'd seen it so many times with women over the years.

There were young girls who were afraid of losing their hair, so they didn't seek medical help with their breasts because of the fear of chemotherapy and what that would do to their hair. I sympathized with the young women, knowing how important hair is in our community, but I tried to stress that any hair lost would grow back. And if it didn't, there were wigs and weaves.

Or the women who didn't go for breast check- because their men are "breast men" and the very idea of losing their breasts was horrifying.

I didn't take the approach of telling anyone that their fears were crazy. I just tried to reassure them that their health should take priority over everything else. And I tried to hammer home that no woman should be afraid of finding out if she has breast cancer. Early detection really does work. And educating your-self can be the difference between life and death.

#MakeHealthATopPriority

CHAPTER 8

GROWING THE DREAM

"So many of our dreams at first seem impossible, then they seem improbable, and then, when we summon the will, they soon become inevitable."

-*Christopher Reeve*

*T*here came a point in my life where I found myself working around the clock, with education and advocacy. And my dream of finding a sisterhood had finally come to fruition.

In September 1994, I started Sisters Network Inc. Like I'd been doing before, I visited churches, support groups and other places to share the news about this new, first-of-its kind organization for black women dealing with breast cancer.

The first Sisters Network meeting was held at the Riverside Clinic in the medical center area of Houston, Texas. We had fifteen survivors show up to that first meeting, representing all ages, backgrounds, and spectrums and we immediately bonded.

Since I didn't have an advertising budget, word of mouth

was what got those women there. We didn't have a formal meeting agenda, so we sat in a circle and shared our testimonies. Women were free to not only talk about their operations, but their personal feelings as well.

During our first support meeting, we adopted this quote to say at each meeting thereafter: "I love you just the way you are," and I incorporated that into our meeting structure. Later, we still preferred to start our meetings with that. We hugged each other and encouraged one another to love each other just as we were.

Our mission was and has not changed: *Sisters Network Inc. is committed to increasing local and national attention to the devastating impact that breast cancer has in the African American community.*

Being part of a support group where the members could look around and see other African American women, gave each a heightened sense of freedom. Every woman could be who she was and feel more comfortable. Sisterhood was about the ability to reach out, and the opportunity to bond. But friendships took time to forge.

We met again a month later and started doing potluck gatherings and inviting guests. Eventually, we pulled our resources together to get programs printed. At that time, I did not know how to use the computer for design, so I'd handwrite the pamphlets and then someone else would type it up.

Our first newsletter debuted in 1995. The early versions were in black and white, as was the logo. My sister reminded me of the time I cut out facial silhouettes and placed the faces in different positions until I decided on two women back to back for the logo. Our current logo reflects that same image I manually created in the beginning.

Many of our members contributed their poetry and photography for newsletter content. Our second newsletter featured a full-length body photograph of an African American woman: half covered, but exposing her post-mastectomy chest with no breast reconstruction. The image was very in-your-face and some churches commented that it was slightly offensive. But at the time, this reality dose was needed in the community to put a tangible face on breast cancer.

In that same issue, Sylvia Dunnavant wrote a poem entitled *Am I Not A Woman?* It is still one of my favorite poems of all-time.

Am I Not A Woman?

My shape has been changed.
My form has been revised.
My breast has been desized.
Am I not a woman?
My heart still loves.
My arms still hug.
My body still craves.
Am I not a woman?
My hips still swerve.
My lips still entice.
My eyes still allure.
Am I not a woman?
My fingers still caress.
My mouth still soothes.
My ears still listen tenderly.
Am I not a woman?

THE POEM TOUCHED me because the poet was communicating that, despite the physical changes of her breasts, she was still a whole woman. A small part of her body had been altered but upon closer inspection, she was the same woman she'd always been. Still able to love, desire, nurture, and listen.

Our first organizational community program was a faith-based initiative. Each member committed to hosting a breast cancer awareness campaign at her respective congregation. We made our own pink ribbons and brochures and enrolled in classes to learn more about breast health.

At the time, many similar organizations functioned locally and there was little uniformity. I knew that in order for our community to progress and stop the silence, we needed a strong united front. We needed to be advocates and we needed a national movement.

We also began our annual Gift of Life Block Walk in which we walked door-to-door in predominantly African American neighborhoods to educate residents about breast health and cancer awareness. Since people weren't coming to us, we were taking the messages to the streets.

I've always considered Sisters Network to be a movement. Sisters Network was established to change the way our people approached breast cancer and these changes would be a direct reaction against the previous generations handling of the disease.

I come from a family of strong community advocates. My mother was wonderful at it. So, I didn't feel like I needed a college degree or a 501(c)3 to start a national organization, but I needed to be a good organizer. I believed in putting all my thoughts on paper and developing a written business plan. Thoughts and ideas were great, but if those thoughts and ideas just bounced around in my head, they may have never come to fruition.

I was determined to set the ball high in motion and believed everything would eventually fall into place.

Our second chapter debuted in Los Angeles, but it failed to sustain at that time. I didn't view this as a failure but rather as an opportunity to improve and identify organizational deficiencies.

While attending a conference on disparities in health care, I was elated to meet other breast cancer survivors from various cities. Although this particular conference was not specific to breast cancer, the women were eager to get together after the conference activities and share experiences and support. I located the conference director and asked if I could have a meeting room. (In 1997, I was receiving the "Hope Award" at this very same conference.) So there I was, calling a meeting at a hotel in Washington, D.C.

The women were so enthusiastic, and since they were at a conference, it was clear they were also hungry for information and committed to the cause. My aim at that time was to be in cities and rural areas where women of color had very little or no support. I didn't want to duplicate successful programs, but rather fill a hole where there were obvious voids.

At this time, breast cancer was still considered a white woman's disease, so when African Americans attended these conferences, all cancers and treatments were addressed unilaterally.

As I sat in that D.C. hotel, I found myself questioning whether there was any residual value to this meeting. It was long before I realized that there was. From this impromptu meeting, I was able to identify a number of strong survivors from different states to work with me in developing new affiliate chapters.

What a wonderful idea it was! A successful and innovative concept that was able to help sisters gain a large foothold on a national basis.

Let me offer encouragement if you have a large vision or if you are feeling discouraged because your dreams aren't growing as fast as you would like, always remember there is hope.

The first advice I would give someone wanting to start a nonprofit organization is to adopt a "can-do" attitude. Your vision will be tested and challenged frequently by naysayers, so you must believe in your vision and yourself. My own mother and daughter didn't initially want me to take on this tremendous task, for different reasons. My immediate family worried that I was taking on too much and needed to rest and relax more. But they soon realized the importance of such an organization. It's imperative that you believe in yourself, in your mission, even if no one else does.

Another step is finding people in your community who are willing to support you by volunteering their time or donating their resources. Sisters Network was so lucky in the incubation stage to find survivors and other people who supported our vision and mission and were willing to donate their time, services, materials and resources.

Lastly, network and build relationships with other agencies and nonprofits that you may be able to partner with. If that organization is already well-established, they can really help your new organization grow. Never be afraid to ask for help. Remember what I've stressed before, no one can help you if they don't know what the problem is.

CHAPTER 9

SISTERS NETWORK INC.

"Is solace anywhere more comforting than that in the arms of a sister."
-Alice Walker

ecause of the noticeable lack of "sisterhood" in the traditional organizations, my mind remained in overdrive on a regular basis: What could I do to help? How could anyone get through this alone, and why should they have to?

Oftentimes, I would get angry – about my situation, about the lack of resources for women of color, because the disease had chosen me. Just angry. And scared. Of the unknown, of worst-case scenarios. Of no longer feeling like me.

But by the time I started Sisters Network, I had reached a point where I decided to turn that anger into strength, and fear into drive and determination.

There would be obstacles, though. Lots of them. I was told that no one would open their door, no one would listen, and no one would care. These were all proven to be wrong over time.

Being a part of an organization like Sisters Network was so critical when trying to manage the full spectrum of emotions that came with a breast cancer diagnosis, the treatment, and recovery. It was comforting to know that none of us were alone.

At the time, Sisters Network was governed by an elected board of directors and assisted by an appointed medical advisory committee. As the organization grew rapidly, I sadly found myself having less time to dedicate to personal one-on-one outreach. Luckily, I had a small dedicated staff and survivor's advocates in place, so I was confident in entrusting daily operations and programs to them.

On any given day, I received dozens of emails from survivors or women who supported our mission. Oftentimes, it was a simple 'thank you for what you do' or it was a request for assistance or information. Some days, it was just not possible to respond to all in a timely manner. That didn't mean that I didn't care or didn't want to help, but there was only so much I, or any one person, could do, which is why I had a great staff in place. Each and every one of those staffers and survivor volunteers were committed to the vision and cause.

In 1999, Sisters Network broke new ground by hosting the nation's first National African American Breast Cancer Conference. The goals of the first conference were "Public education regarding early cancer detection, motivation, and training of community leaders to implement screenings at home with a focus on breast cancer and African Americans." This message seems so simple now, but it was critical at that time.

The first conference was held at the Marriott West Loop Hotel in Houston and offered more than ten workshops including Importance of Clinical Trials, Breast Self-Examination Training, Overcoming Cultural Barriers to Effective Cancer Screening Programs and Alternative Mental Health Strategies for Healing through Breast Cancer. All of these topics are still very relevant all these years later.

Subsequent conferences have focused on replacing FEAR with HOPE and empowering women through positive educational messages. The national annual three-day conference offers CEU and CHES accreditation and is attended by survivors, breast cancer experts, legislators, and healthcare professionals, and provides a venue for Sisters Network membership to partner with other supporting entities.

Sisters celebrated their tenth anniversary at the national African American Breast Cancer conference in October of 2009. This particular conference was a milestone, which bares special mention since we had survived that long. The conference attracted more than five hundred attendees, including nationally recognized medical experts and was held in large metropolitan cities such as Houston, Chicago, Atlanta, Richmond, and Detroit. Every year I looked forward to the conference because I also celebrated another year of survivorship and, like the participants, I shared in their excitement and always left inspired and recharged.

Several of the attendees were only able to attend on scholarship and we were very grateful for the pharmaceutical companies and corporate sponsors that underwrote those scholarships so that women could not only receive emotional support, but have access to the latest information and medical advancements concerning their health.

At that point, we ran the organization out of my apartment. My husband and I retreated to the back of the apartment and my staff set up shop in the front. The residential management was very supportive of what we were doing. I was not going to let lack of office space stop me from my mission.

In 2006, SNI launched the Raising the House campaign dedicated to raising funds for the Sister House initiative. We wanted a sanctuary for breast cancer survivors to bond, hold meetings and events, and receive much-needed support services.

We were finally able to break ground on Sister House and the day of the ribbon-cutting was one of my proudest moments. More than one hundred guests, mostly survivors, attended the event dressed in their pink attire. Sister House was my dream come true. My vision was to create a comfortable "home away from home" for patients, survivors, families, and the community.

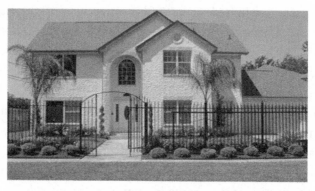

Sisters Network Sister House/National Headquarters
-Houston, Texas
Circa 2008-2018

SISTERS HOUSE SAT APPROXIMATELY two miles from M.D. Anderson Cancer Center and centrally located in mid-Third Ward, a historic Houston community with an underserved population. We had a partnership with local housing suites that assisted patients receiving treatment with a free shuttle to the medical center, complimentary hot breakfast, and complimentary airport shuttle.

In addition to serving as the national headquarters, there was a full kitchen, computer lab, and resource library.

The national office provided standardized outreach programs (which are implemented today by the affiliate chapters), breast health education collateral materials, community educational forums, and clinical trial recruitment assistance to major studies. Additionally, we collaborated with various organizations and corporate partners to increase breast cancer awareness in urban communities.

My purpose in life made every day meaningful. I loved helping other survivors meet their needs because I truly didn't want any woman to feel like she had to be alone on this journey. Every time I drove up to Sister House, I got a renewed sense of pride and accomplishment. It was everything that I always envisioned it to be. Each room had been carefully decorated with items donated from various Sisters Network chapters and provided a feeling of comfort, relaxation and support. It was important for the national headquarters to physically represent who we were as an organization and a people.

"[WHILE IN HOUSTON], I got to see the pink house. Tears come to my eyes and I get chills when I think of where you came from and where you are now."

-Excerpt from email from
Sisters supporter Pam

WE HAD to sell the house in 2018 because it just became too hard to manage, but the work of Sisters Network continues.

We currently have a national board of eight carefully selected members. Our national outreach programs include a Pink Ribbon Awareness Initiative, Gift for Life Block Walk, and our first annual Stop the Silence® walk, which occurred in April 2010. The walk benefits our Breast Cancer Assistance Program (BCAP), which provides assistance to women facing financial challenges after diagnosis. This program has been in existence since late 2006 and has provided financial assistance for mammograms, rent, office visits, prescriptions, medical related lodging, and transportation. Funds raised from the Stop the Silence walk will continue to assist women throughout the United States.

Much of my day now is spent serving as a resource for clinical trial and focus group recruitment, participating in medical conference calls, serving as a liaison and communicating between medical organizations and black breast cancer patients and survivors; many of whom I have never even met. I personally make an attempt to respond to every woman who reaches out to me during her treatment but we do have systems in place to provide greater service and outreach through our volunteer network.

I really look forward our annual sister training retreats. Our most recent retreat was a first-of-its-kind two-and-a-half day retreat held in Memphis, Tennessee, with ninety-four members in attendance including staff, chapter presidents and vice presidents, and associate members. We completed a research questionnaire for a major university that will help produce an educational awareness video aimed at early detection. Prior to our involvement, many of these educational videos lacked an African American component.

The retreats reinspire and reiterate what the organization is about. It is very important for me to encourage my leaders to grow and develop as leaders. I want everyone to be consistent in how meetings are held and how leaders conduct themselves.

When I reflect back on that first Sisters meeting at Riverside Clinic in Houston, Texas, with fifteen women in attendance, I am amazed at the growth of the organization. SNI is nationally recognized as the leading voice and the only national African American breast cancer survivorship organization in the United States.

We have ongoing special events and activities aimed at getting sister members out of the house during treatment and to the point where they won't focus on their pain. There is great comfort in being around those who are going through or have been through the same challenges. Our events are filled with so much love, camaraderie, and encouragement.

SNI also recognizes that breast cancer is a global issue. Global statistics from 2002 indicated there were more than one million new cases of breast cancer. Today, there are more than four million women living with the disease worldwide. By 2021, researchers anticipate there will be twenty million men, women, and children cancer survivors in the U.S.

Sisters Network was also a partner with AACI - Africa Cancer Care Inc. Africa Cancer Care was founded in 2005 as a result of the looming cancer predictions for Africa by the World Health Organization and other international health bodies.

Programs to reduce breast cancer mortality should emphasize the role of routine mammography screening to detect breast cancer at earlier, more treatable stages.

Many African American women are diagnosed at a later stage when tumors are larger and have spread to other parts of the body. Therefore, getting women in earlier for first time screenings and annual mammograms, raising awareness through outreach education in the community, and ongoing collaboration with other community groups is a primary focus of our mobile mammography program.

SNI currently has a presence in twenty-two states with forty-three affiliate chapters. We have affiliate chapters in California, Delaware, Florida, Georgia, Illinois, Indiana, Louisiana, Maryland, Michigan, Mississippi, Nebraska, New Jersey, New York, North Carolina, Ohio, Oklahoma, South Carolina, Tennessee, Texas, Virginia, and Wisconsin.

SNI continues to develop new chapters and expand the

national outreach through its affiliate survivor run chapters nationwide.

At the core of Sisters Network mission is support, outreach and education. During 2019, Sisters breast health outreach initiatives impacted an estimated 1.9 million families through chapter outreach, television, radio and print media.

The organization's trademark and successful national community outreach programs include: "The Gift For Life Block Walk" and "The Pink Ribbon Awareness Project." These initiatives are implemented through the Sisters Network affiliate chapters.

As the survivorship movement emerges, guidelines are being developed for survivor care beyond the basics of making healthy lifestyle choices. Many patients are experiencing post-traumatic stress disorder (PTSD). Continuously thinking about the cancer, restlessness, insomnia, and panic attacks have all been reported post-treatment. True healing goes beyond the medical treatment. For some women, lifestyle choices may not be enough.

As survivors, I believe that we must continue to evolve. Never underestimate your power as a survivor. Survivor advocates play a critical role in the oncology population as they are powerful and trusted members. They serve as ambassadors, guidance counselors, and healthcare monitors. Survivors can always be heard on Capitol Hill using their voice and testimonies to incite change and protect funds for cancer research. Survivors with a working knowledge of breast cancer have a great advantage when it comes to helping others along the journey.

On my cancer journey, I was extremely blessed to have had such a tight-knit family who took hold of the situation and led me. But I began to wonder and sympathize with the women who did not have that type of family support, insurance, or even financial support. I had a rough time with all the advantages I had and couldn't imagine how someone else could cope with such a disadvantage.

Every survivor needs someone around her to guide her and encourage her on the journey. With Sisters Network, no one has to take this journey alone.

CHAPTER 10

FROM THE SIDELINES TO THE HEADLINES

"My mission in life is not merely to survive, but to thrive; and to do so with some passion, some compassion, some humor, and some style."
-Maya Angelou

*A*s a CEO of a nationally recognized organization, I am still in awe of the lives that Sisters Network touches every day, whether it is through our chapter's survivor's work and national outreach initiatives or providing funds via our breast cancer assistance program, or assisting survivors and providing free mammograms to those who are uninsured or underinsured.

In 2006, we started the BCAP program, a financial assistance program that's geared to helping survivors with financial challenges, like rent and utilities, etc.

The program provided $100,000 in financial support to survivors in 2018, even during a very difficult transitional time for Sisters Network. We were losing members and the organization was struggling financially.

In 2020, when the Coronavirus pandemic hit, we added money for groceries to the BCAP program. We also help women who need mammograms and ultrasounds who are not survivors. So, the two-pronged program helps the community and helps survivors.

All too often, I would receive a call that we had lost another sister to breast cancer. It saddened me and it saddened our organization. However, it also inspired me and all of our members to keep going in the fight against breast cancer.

The black woman's breast cancer struggle is our story, our lives and our legacy. Our commitment to serving the African American community and providing exceptional support resources and financial assistance is who we are as a sisterhood organization.

Hundreds of interviews, television appearances, and print articles have featured Sisters Network and with each media hit, we raise awareness of who we are and what we do. The media has an obligation, in my opinion, to continue to provide information on breast cancer and provide an accurate face on black breast cancer.

Several young women who were diagnosed with late stage breast cancer said that the reason they waited so long to see a doctor was because they just didn't realize that women who looked like them could get the disease. Particularly, with the urban media, they should be charged with socially responsible news reporting and health updates.

In December 2009, Sisters Network was honored by the Africa Cancer Care, Inc. (ACCI) organization. The organization is comprised of a group of individuals devoted to bridging cancer care disparities in the United States and Africa. I was presented with the award during their annual ACCI banquet and awards ceremony. Her Excellency, Mrs. Turai Yar'Adua, the then First Lady of the Federal Republic of Nigeria, was in attendance for the special event. I was extremely honored to receive this award and look forward to more global partnerships. Our work at Sisters Network should not be limited to black women in the United States. Our sisters in Africa also need to learn about breast health and the importance of early detection.

I was honored to be featured on the cover of *Breast Cancer Wellness* magazine, a national publication. In the article entitled "Sisters Network: Making a Difference to Stop the Silence," I discussed the evolution of Sisters Network and the importance of women putting their health first. We were also profiled in 2009 in the *Fort Bend Journal* where we discussed the work of the organization and our plans to start a Fort Bend area affiliate chapter in the Houston area, one of the county's largest African American populations. I have so much passion and commitment for educating my sisters around the nation. I am dedicated to changing our story to a celebration of life. We've accomplished so much over the last fifteen years, but there is still so much work to be done. I'm not interested in a brick and mortar building in every major city. I am interested in a cure.

As I reflect on the many accomplishments of sisters networking over the 27 years of survivorship, my heart stays full with joy and peace. I think of the lifesaving breast cancer outreach work that our national network of African American breast cancer survivors continues to provide each and every day. I am truly humbled and honored to be in the company of my sisters.

Our affiliate membership base friends and family have worked tirelessly to lay a strong foundation for our organization. Even through financial challenges by traditional transitional changes, we still form new community partnerships, expanding outreach initiatives, creating new national initiatives, and continuing to take our leadership and advocacy work to the next level.

Sisters Network is fortunate and grateful that, even though our various streams of financial and volunteer support have been diminished, we continue to focus on our very important national mission of educating African American women about the devastating impact of breast cancer and saving lives.

Our work is making a difference. I see it in the women that approach me. I read about it in the hundreds of emails we get. A woman approached me who had heard of Sisters Network. She was scared because she didn't have health insurance. I just happened to have an opportunity to go onto a radio program to talk about Sisters Network, and I shared this woman's story. We were attempting to raise money to help her cover the cost of treatment. An anonymous donor contacted us to pay for her treatment.

This was a wonderful but unusual story. Really, every day we have success stories. We are out there talking to women in our community about breast health, helping the newly diagnosed, and providing support to long-term survivors. We're providing the education that is needed and also connecting to resources.

It's important for women to learn about available and appropriate resources and how to access them within their communities. Some people may think that if they get sick, they can go to the local hospital and the doctors can help them heal. But not all hospitals are equipped to handle cancer. Not all cities have a cancer center. We believe that there are people within the African American community who have breast cancer and insurance, yet don't know how to go about finding the best care available. You should be seen by a doctor who specializes in your type of cancer. Anytime we can ensure one more woman is aware of the best resources and care available to her, well, that is a success.

I was recently in San Antonio for the International Breast Cancer Conference. It's the largest conference on breast cancer in the world. Out of thousands of people there, there were less than 30 black women.

So, I try to take the knowledge I have garnered in those

settings and share with the support groups that we are connected to so that the women aren't left out.

One of the areas where I would love to see growth, is having more soldiers on the battlefield. Prior to 2020, we had not been able to move forward on making policy changes because there were not enough women who are interested in advocacy. You have to show up. You have to go to Washington. You have to talk to your Congressmen or Congresswomen or your Senator. But we couldn't seem to get a large enough number of women who wanted to be a part of that process.

We are now, however, inspired by the recent shift in mindset toward advocacy. We're still at a point as a community where we're trying to accept the fact that we have the worst outcome of breast cancer. We need advocates fighting on our behalf.

Our numbers are dismal in the advancing policy part because we lack knowledge and training. The other part is some in the medical policy industry simply don't care enough to include participants who look like us or have our best interests at heart.

PART II
Here we go
again...

CHAPTER 11

SECOND, THIRD & FOURTH TIME AROUND

"When things are bad, we take comfort in the thought that they could always get worse. And when they are, we find hope in the thought that things are so bad they have to get better."
-Malcolm Forbes

*T*he only thing worse than getting breast cancer is getting breast cancer AGAIN.

And in my case, again. And again.

That's right. While I was building Sisters Network, working hard on behalf of others and celebrating my own health accomplishments, cancer reared its ugly head again.

I've been diagnosed with breast cancer three times since 1993 and the last three times have been DCIS (ductal carcinoma in situ), the early stage, pre-cancer and DCIS infiltrating.

If you're going to have a breast cancer incident, you'd like it to be at DCIS stage. If you do not find it at that stage, it will go to the next stage, then the next, and the next. So, it's imperative to be in tune with your body. I mention that throughout this book because I can't say it often enough.

I feel very blessed that the previous times I had cancer, I had educated myself so that I could actually show my oncologist where I felt the cancer, not with using my fingers, but by feeling the sensation inside.

Since 1993, I've had both my mammogram and my ultrasound. The standard protocol offered includes getting a mammogram, but I learned early on that the mammogram was not enough to find cancer. You need both a mammogram and an ultrasound. That was why as an organization, Sisters Network always encouraged women to make sure they annually got mammograms and ultrasounds.

Prior to my fourth diagnosis, I had my mammogram and my ultrasound, as normal. The results came back fine. But I knew my body and something didn't feel right; something was wrong. The sensation was back again. Thank God that I was at MD Anderson and my doctor didn't question me when I suggested an MRI. She just ordered it. I'd been with her for many years, so she knew that I knew my body.

She ordered the MRI and lo and behold, the cancer was there. It had not been detected by the mammogram or the ultrasound. Think about it. For me as an individual and as a CEO of a national organization for breast cancer, it was troubling that while number one, I had that experience. Number two, I knew the protocol, I'm glad I had the wherewithal to know that it wasn't enough to find this fourth cancer.

What I've endured would be enough to break the strongest of souls. And I'm not going to lie, sometimes I felt broken. But I was not giving up.

I believe that one's determination and the ability to rally yourself is crucial. Even if no one else does, you can rally yourself to do some things you never thought you could do.

What makes this even harder is there is an array of emotions that you go through in the roller coaster of recurring breast cancer. Each stage is a different sphere.

Of course, once you've been diagnosed, you're concerned about having metastatic breast cancer, which means it has spread from your breast to another part of your body. That's that's the greatest fear once you're diagnosed. That's a different fear from when you are waiting to find out if you even have breast cancer.

I could say that my greatest fear now is the fact that my cancer wasn't found with the standardized method. Everyone can't get an MRI every year because it's too expensive, so this is a very real problem.

Breast cancer recurrence is something that makes people uncomfortable, afraid and reluctant to even think about. The five-year post-diagnosis mark is a desired milestone, but it is not always a permanent green light. It's a grim reality but breast cancer may reoccur in the same breast, the other breast or in a different organ. And just when you feel like your life is returning to some sense of normalcy, a second diagnosis rears its ugly head; turning your life upside down. You may begin to question your treatment, wondering if you and your doctor did everything you could do to fight the cancer. You may even feel hopeless.

Research has not been able to pinpoint any direct causes of why one patient may remain in remission for years and another patient who underwent the same treatment protocol may experience a recurrence. Breast cancer, like all cancer, is unpredictable and you may find yourself overwhelmed by fears that it will happen again.

Separation anxiety post-treatment is normal. Many survivors report that they miss the constant interaction and attention they received during treatment and it's a difficult shift back to "normal" life. Remember to be proud of what you have achieved by completing the grueling treatments and completing your plan of action.

Some survivors may find that joining a support group (online or in person) may help them share their fears and hopes with other survivors who truly understand what they are going through or feeling.

Approximately twenty percent of all survivors will experience a recurrence. Just like an initial diagnosis, it is critical to catch the new cancer at an early stage to have a better outcome. Work closely with your medical team to determine the best approach for the best outcome. Remember that you will be more familiar with what to expect the second or subsequent times around. The same strength and resources you drew from during your initial battle can be the same ones that help you through the second or any subsequent battles.

There's also the issue of medication. At the 2009 San Antonio Breast Cancer Symposium, one of the findings addressed was whether Herceptin was more effective if given with chemotherapy. Taking the drug (trastuzumab) helped more women live longer without a recurrence, new research found. Other symposium topics included finding the right hormonal therapy combination, adding Avastin may slow disease progression and Denosumab outperforms Zometa in treating bone mestases. (Please clear any medication with your own doctor, I simply want to give you insight into what I've discovered in my research).

There are some things you can do to minimize your recurrence risk, including adopting a healthier lifestyle, which means controlling your weight, increasing your exercise and limiting tobacco and alcohol use. Don't stop doing your monthly breast exams and continue to be the biggest advocate for your own health.

Learn to get in touch with what makes you happy! Laughing releases endorphins that improve mood and feel-good brain chemicals. Make time for things that bring you joy even if you have to schedule activities for yourself. And most importantly, relax. Don't spend time worrying about things you can't change.

Facing cancer a second or subsequent time requires strength and hope. It is normal to feel angry and fearful but remember that you don't have to be alone. Sisters Network has members who are two, even three time survivors and we can help pair you up with a sister mentor to help ease the process.

CHAPTER 12

NEVER GIVE UP

"You may encounter many defeats, but you must not be defeated. In fact, it may be necessary to encounter the defeats, so you can know who you are, what you can rise from, how you can still come out of it."
-Maya Angelou

*B*y the time my cancer returned, I had been involved in the breast cancer area for many, many years. My attitude about the recurrence took on a matter-of-fact mentality, rather than fear and paralysis. I had done that and had no intention of repeating it because taking control and educating myself is what helped save my life.

I have never taken the approach that I *beat* breast cancer. I never approached it with an "I'm cured" frame of mind. My desire was to know all I could to be in tune with my body, reach other African American women and encourage them to walk past fear and go straight to action.

Finding my fourth cancer the way I did (through the MRI) tells me that my work as a leader of an African American breast cancer organization, is still sorely needed.

I recognize that an MRI, even if you have insurance, is very expensive. So, we're now in the process of researching how many women and what kind of research is out there recommending MRI in addition to ultrasounds and mammograms. And so far, we have found very little information. I know that I can't have been that unusual in having the MRI show that I had two new cancers. That's why it's imperative that we either find the research, or request additional research because women can die from doing what they think is just standard, normal protocol (mammogram and ultrasound).

That means, my fight rages on.

And in the midst of the war, my personal battle rages on. I am taking a chemotherapy pill every day. And yes, I have minor reactions to it. Nothing major and so far, I haven't seen any adverse reactions. I've seen some changes, but nothing that I can't handle. So my overall health and my results, in general, have been very good. In that regard, I am blessed.

In fact, I'm actually blessed in so many ways. I've always been a dedicated fighter. Battling breast cancer proved that even more and showed me how it's imperative that you never give up.

And as bleak as it may seem to you or your loved one suffering from breast cancer, it's imperative that you don't give up either.

If you're not involved with an organization, or up on your reading, or attending conferences, you will not be able to help yourself. You have to be your own best advocate and we help you learn how to be an advocate not only for yourself because it's necessary, but for your family, your friends and colleagues. Knowledge is power and the power that you gain from organizations like Sisters Network will be with you forever.

And then, once you've educated yourself, do not keep it to yourself. Be an advocate for your community. As survivors, we can tell our story to help the next person going to go through breast cancer. Each story is different. Each of us has different lives and have chosen different paths. So your journey, even though you may have the same diagnosis, is your complete and individual experience. That's why your experience must be shared.

Remember how scared I said I was when I was initially diagnosed? How I was not able to fully comprehend or think about what I needed to do next? That's one of the reasons why I believe that Sisters Network is so important to all women. No matter what stage you are diagnosed, no matter how much money you have in the bank or in your purse, no matter how much education or family support you have, you, as an individual, need to be able to say to someone what the next step is.

This is a lifetime journey. This cancer is not something you are diagnosed with, you get better, and it's over. How I wish that were true, but it is not. You have to stay in the movement, stay alert, stay active, and be your own best advocate in order to help the next one. You must stay involved in the movement of breast cancer so that collectively as a network, we can help make a difference in policy and in how our community moves toward action.

It's why even if you're healed, your work is never done.

CHAPTER 13

MY SISTER, MY FRIEND

"Sisterhood is magical and medicinal - use it as a lifelong resource."
-Claudia Black

hen I think of the female bonds forged within Sisters Network, it warms my heart. Not only does being among a legion of sisters give us a "safe space," it allows women to regain their truth, confidence, and support for one another.

Sisters stay strong and are a cohesive unit. They are a source of tough but unconditional love. Simply put, a sister sacrifices, encourages, forgives, and inspires. It is a tight bond that should never be broken.

I asked a few women what sisterhood meant to them.

"Sisters bring out the best in me."

"My sister is my favorite person to be around."

"I can go to my sister when I'm in a tight spot."

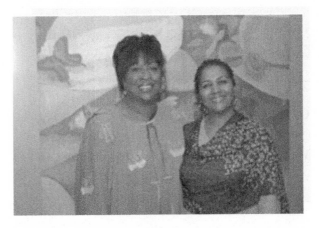

My sister Kim and I

IN 2001, my sister Kim wrote our national poem *Stop the Silence*. Inspired by our family history of breast cancer and reluctance by our elders to discuss it openly, the poem asserts our mission to fight breast cancer and stop the silence.

I'm elated to share it with you on the next page:

STOP THE SILENCE, hear our cry.
Mo more need to pass us by.
We're mothers and sisters and some brothers too.
We're just trying to get the word out to you.

STOP THE SILENCE, we know the challenge is great.
We won't be silent, you know lives are at stake.
We're spreading the word as we go door to door.
We're marching for justice,
and we won't be ignored.

STOP THE SILENCE, we won't give up.
Our body may be weak, but our soul is tough.
If you look at our faces, we are the same.
We're standing united, no longer ashamed.

STOP THE SILENCE, our gloves are on.
We're fighting breast cancer,
our commitment is strong!
Pledge hours of service, your money or time.
Let's fight this together, that's the bottom line.

So, STOP THE SILENCE, the hour is NOW!
We're building partnerships,
and we'll tell you how.
All we need is commitment, so what do you say?
We're stating our case and we're marching today.

Stop the Silence.
Just Stop the Silence.
Oh, STOP . . . the Silence TODAY.

ALL THESE YEARS LATER, that poem warms my heart. Not just because the words resonate with me, but because I felt the love from my sister.

But what I also learned is that true sisterhood can run just as deep as blood. My best friend, Yvonne, and I have been friends for more than forty-five years. We both grew up in New Jersey, but fate would have us meet when we were both living in Los Angeles. I was going through a divorce at the time and Yvonne's friendship was very much welcomed. I can't stress enough the importance of female friendships when life presents a challenge.

"REGARDLESS OF OUR DIFFERENCES, we have remained focused on our friendship. Our love for each other is stronger than anything that could divide us."

- Yvonne

THE PREMISE behind Sisters Network is to create a sisterhood of support and caregiving. Caregivers can be family, friends, neighbors, colleagues or volunteers. Caregivers play a crucial role in survivor recovery but remember, caregivers must learn ways to take care of themselves too. While giving care, it's normal to put your own needs and feelings aside, but this is not good for your overall well-being and health. You need to take care of yourself, too. If you're not taking care of yourself, you can't take care of anyone else. Think about it: If you let your portable battery delete its charge, it's incapable of charging anything else.

You may not like to think of yourself as a caregiver because you are caring for someone you love, and doing that act seems natural. You may find that you even share the emotional roller coaster with your loved one. This is common, but if the feelings become overwhelming, you should reach out and talk to a counselor or social worker.

I consider the sisterhood the foundation of our organization. We're sisters. We're friends. We're a family of sisterhood, and we live by the premise that you can count on your family to uplift you, to walk with you, to guide you, to be there at your darkest point and to share your happiest point. We try to strive to find the new normal that as survivors adjusting to our situation as it evolves once diagnosed, is not something that you say, I've rung the bell, it's finished. 'I have nothing else to think about or be concerned about.'

Having been a breast cancer survivor, this type of disease of cancer, it follows you each and every day. It is a challenge and is a challenge that we all can win, but it is not easy, and we all need each other to help us understand to keep updated with the constant changes within the movement and the arena of breast cancer.

Here are some resources to help you along the way:

FAMILY CAREGIVER ALLIANCE
Support for families and friends who are caregivers
Phone: 1-800-445-8106
Web site: www.caregiver.org

NATIONAL FAMILY CAREGIVERS Association
Information, education, and support for caregivers
Phone: 1-800-896-3650
Web site: www.nfcacares.org

CHAPTER 14

THE UNIQUE CHALLENGES WE FACE

"When we least expect it, life sets us a challenge to test our courage and willingness to change."

-Paulo Coelho

*A*frican American survivors have a unique set of challenges when treating breast cancer. In fact, I've found that we have more recovery challenges post-diagnosis.

A nursing study conducted at The University of Pittsburgh Nursing School concluded that low-income African American women uniquely experienced greater physical and social distress and more uncertainty about treatment and treatment goals than the other delineated racial and economic groups. Chronic levels of stress may affect cancer risks and promote unhealthy habits such as overeating, smoking, drug use and alcohol abuse. Survivors also report nightmares, irritability, anxiety, insomnia, and ignoring subsequent health signs.

Black breast cancer patients have a unique set of challenges and those challenges increase after being diagnosed more than other groups of women.

One major medical concern is that black women have

increased rates of "triple negative" breast cancer (TNBC) - rare tumors that are not driven by estrogen, progesterone or a mutation in the Her-2 gene. These tumors are particularly difficult to treat because they do not respond to certain therapies (such as Tamoxifen and Aromatase inhibitors), which have been helpful in preventing breast cancer recurrences.

Most disturbingly, one of the statistics I mentioned earlier: black women are less likely to get breast cancer but more likely to die. That is really something to think about.

Education and knowledge will continue to erode long-held fears and superstitions in the black community; a fact that researchers increasingly believe has at least as much to do with biology as with access to health care and screening tools like mammography.

African American women are less likely than white women to get a mammogram because of problems with access to them and because healthcare providers are less likely to refer African American women for mammograms. Studies have found that when African-American and white women use mammography equally, breast cancer is diagnosed in them at similar stages.

Ninety percent of white women who are diagnosed with breast cancer will live at least five years, but only seventy-six percent of black women with breast cancer will live five years, according to the American Cancer Society (ACS). Five years is considered a pivotal marker for long-term cancer survival.

The breast cancer death rate of elderly black women increased in the first half of the 1990s in the U.S., even though the death rate among white women declined during the same period. The increase is especially puzzling because until 1993, the rate of breast cancer deaths was lower in black women aged seventy and older than in elderly white women. Several studies have shown that during the 1970s and 1980s, even though the death rate from breast cancer in younger women was higher in blacks than in whites, older black women were less likely than older white women to die from breast cancer.

But some research indicates that death rates from breast cancer declined in whites, but not in blacks, during the first half of the 1990s. In fact, from 1993 to 1996, the breast cancer death rate in women aged thirty-five and younger was more than twice as high in blacks than in whites.

Triple-negative tumors are also fast growing and have an early risk of recurrence in the first three to five years after diagnosis as opposed to cancers expressing hormone receptors. Triple negative breast cancer has one of the worst prognoses of any other breast cancer because it is unresponsive to the most effective treatments for breast cancer. Triple negative breast cancer represents approximately fifteen percent of breast cancer cases in the United States. European researchers conclude that patients with triple negative status are no more likely to relapse or die of breast cancer than patients with other receptor profiles. However, when relapse occurs, it tends to be earlier and subsequent death sooner than other receptor groups. Therefore, triple-negative patients may benefit from careful and early follow-up after breast cancer treatment.

Dr. Joyce O'Shaughnessy, co-director of breast cancer research at Baylor Charles A. Sammons Cancer Center at Dallas, says that many patients see a diagnosis of triple-negative as a death sentence.

"That's not the case at all. Many patients are cancer-free many years after treatment," O'Shaughnessy said.

The doctor also points out that the disease recurs within five years after diagnosis in about thirty-two percent of patients compared with only around fifteen percent of patients with other breast cancer types. The chance of recurrence highlights the need for more effective treatment.

Sisters Network Chief Medical Advisor Dr. Lisa Newman has traveled to Ghana to conduct research on TNBC. Dr.

Newman collaborates with doctors in Kumasi, Ghana, in hopes of discovering the origins of the aggressive and difficult to treat form of breast cancer. According to the ACS, triple negative breast cancer represents approximately fifteen percent of breast cancer cases in the United States.

Between the unusual tumors and the fact that black women are more likely than white women to get breast cancer at a young age, researchers say genetics almost definitely plays an important role in the higher death rate among African Americans. Identifying the biological reasons behind the death rate isn't an easy task. Most national studies into breast cancer are focused on white women; mostly because white women are more likely to participate in a study. Also, many of these trials and big studies have a preponderance of white women of a certain economic level and we really need to look at advocating for more women of color to be evaluated. It's only recently that researchers have started studies to look specifically at black women and other minorities, and it takes time to build those studies and get measurable results from them. In the meantime, public health officials need to focus even more resources on educating black women and their families about early diagnosis and making sure they get the best treatment available.

Experts agree that genetics is the next frontier. A University of Chicago 2005 study found that genetic mutations in the breast cancer susceptibility genes (BRCA1 and BRCA2)occur with "appreciable frequency" in African American women with a family history of the disease, with more than one quarter testing positive for a mutation in one of these genes that indicates high risk. Future strategies may involve genetic testing to individualize patient treatment and even techniques to repair or replace harmful genes before breast cancer occurs. However, rapidly expanding medical knowledge can also leave women feeling overwhelmed as they grapple with practical treatment decisions.

CHAPTER 15

HEALTH CARE: WHOM CAN YOU TRUST?

*"Few things help an individual more than to place responsibility upon
him, and to let him know that you trust him."*
-Booker T. Washington

For most cancers, African Americans have the highest cancer mortality rates and the worst survival rates of any population. Black women are less likely to develop breast cancer yet have the highest age-adjusted mortality rates from breast cancer of any racial/ethnic group in the United States. African American women have poorer survival rates than their white and Hispanic counterparts regardless of whether they receive radiation therapy following lumpectomy or mastectomy. Black women, Hispanic women, and poor women were almost fifty percent more likely to experience a longer than six-week gap before radiotherapy treatment which heightens the risk of cancer recurrence.

Experts say that one of the main reasons for this mortality disparity is that black women are diagnosed at more advanced stages of the disease. In other words, we wait too long to seek treatment. Even with this information, for some strange reason black women do not have breast cancer on their mind. In fact, there remains a critical unmet need for basic breast cancer education among black women.

"Stop the Silence" is our national slogan for a reason. It acknowledges the historical inclination of people of color to distrust and decline medical intervention. There is so much basic breast cancer information available in the media but unlike most women, I did think it applied to me.

Prior to my own diagnosis, all of the pamphlets and litera- ture I read had images of older Caucasian women. This misleading face of breast cancer contributes to our lack of knowledge about the risks and symptoms. I strongly feel that the media has an obligation to put a "real" face on health stories and often fail to do so but society must also do its part.

I would encourage more women to be resourceful when it comes to finding answers or solutions that involve their overall health, wellness, and well-being.

At Sisters Network, we receive a lot of assistance requests regarding survivors needing help long after the fact, but we can't fix what we don't know about.

I heard this phrase from a speaker at a conference once and it really resonates with me: 'Often, we assume that people know what we need and when we need it when the reality is that we never expressed to anyone that we needed help.'

No one will come if you don't ask.

African Americans make up less than five percent of physi- cians in this country, according to the American Medical Asso- ciation. Although some racial injustices remain in the healthcare industry, this by no mean is a license not to be responsible for one's health.

Breast cancer is a disease that often strikes a woman in the prime of her life. It attempts to rob her of the very things that define her femininity. Women fear that once they lose their breasts, they lose their womanhood. One does not delight in thinking about illness and disease. As a culture, illness, and disease are something we will deny, ignore, turn it over to God, or seek to blame others. All these excuses lead to high mortality rate in the black community involving serious health matters.

Another obstacle is our genuine distrust of the health care system. Distrust of the health care system is relatively high in the general U.S. population. We can hypothesize that a person's past experiences influences that person's present level of trust. Negative experiences result in a lower level of trust. A patient who has experienced racism or discrimination from individuals and institutions would be less willing to be vulnerable and place trust in a system of unknowns such as medical care. In understanding the role that trust and distrust play in the patient-physician relationship, it's imperative to know that trust is essential to improving the quality of care and in seeking to understand healthcare seeking behaviors across racial/ethnic groups.

Recent analyses of the relationships of minority patients with their physicians have demonstrated that provider racism and patient awareness of past events such as the medical experimentation on slaves and the Tuskegee syphilis experiment have contributed to minority patients having less access to and knowledge of specific medical treatments than their white counterparts, lower levels of trust, and greater unwillingness to participate in clinical trials. Our general mistrust of the health care system has been shaped from the Tuskegee experiment and passed down.

On the other side of the patient-doctor relationship, some worry that a history of distrust of the medical establishment among members of the black community may also be affecting patients' medical decision-making.

The fear factor of going to the doctor is killing us and can result in delaying critical medical screenings. How we can beat breast cancer is to take control of our breast health and overcome our fears of medical treatment! If you have no knowledge, are not persistent and don't follow up, you're not going to be here. It's that simple.

Sisters Network has built and earned the trust of the African American community by our service and support over a quarter of a century.

Disparities in breast cancer survival and treatment for African American and low-income women are well documented yet poorly understood.

Dr. Otis Brawle, former Chief Medical Officer for the American Cancer Society said, "African American women with insurance often do not receive the same level of care as their Caucasian counterparts, and we must work to improve care and outcomes among this population. The black/white survival gap didn't exist before 1981 but since then the disparity has widened."

Researchers have asked whether the cause is biology, environmental or a combination of both. They have also discovered key ways the disease impacts black women. Their cancers are often diagnosed in later staging and they are more likely to have a form of triple negative breast cancer.

And adding poverty to the equation exacerbates the fear factor, says noted scientist Dr. Harold P. Freeman, former president and CEO of New York's North General Hospital, past president of the American Cancer Society and former chairman of the U.S. President's Cancer Panel.

"It's worse when you're afraid and you also don't have knowledge and you don't have insurance and you don't have money," Dr. Freeman said.

A major factor affecting breast cancer survival is the continuing impact of racism in determining who survives. Dr. Freeman says some doctors have been practicing a drive-by diagnosis equivalent to "racial profiling," a "subtle bias in treatment," where black and white people who present the same symptoms receive different treatment. We are seeing each other through the lens of race and making assumptions that are sometimes harmful or even fatal.

The health care choices that people make are clearly a reflection of their social circumstances. There has been evidence showing that physicians' perception of the patient may be affected by race; this includes perceptions of patient's ability to understand choices, a sense of association with patients and the ability to engage patients in their healthcare choices.

Some women, especially black women and older women, may think of doctors as such an intimidating authoritative figure that they are afraid to ask questions out of fear of sounding stupid.

Learn to arrive prepared at your doctor visits. Go to the library, search on the Internet, write down questions and come prepared to see your doctor. You have to train yourself to be your best advocate. I can't say that enough.

According to a National Assessment of Adult Literacy study, only twelve percent of all adults demonstrated proficiency at understanding complex health information. The survey was the federal government's first attempt at quantifying levels of health literacy; the ability of patients to obtain, process, and understand the concepts and medical terms crucial to making informed medical decisions. Even people with advanced degrees still face health literacy challenges.

When African American women are treated for breast cancer, they may be less likely than white women to receive state-of-the-art diagnosis and treatment for breast cancer. This may be influenced by the standard of care in the hospitals where they are treated (smaller hospitals and clinics versus large hospitals and cancer centers) or the existence of racial injustice.

If breast cancer is properly diagnosed, treatment options vary and do not necessarily involve the loss of the breast. The American Cancer Society says that at one time mastectomy was the standard therapy, but now only a percentage of women choose this treatment. The combination of radiation and lumpectomy is much more common today. In many cases, chemotherapy and/or hormonal therapy are also used effectively. But sadly, those options don't seem to be getting through to many black women patients.

The prevailing supposition is that black women are more likely than their white counterparts to die of breast cancer or other cancers related to their reproductive organs. The key is determining if these disparities are caused by societal factors or if black women are genetically predisposed to higher incidences of more aggressive and hard-to-treat cancers.

"African American women tend to get breast-conserving procedures less than the Caucasian population," says National Medical Association spokesperson Dr. Doris Browne, although research indicates that the lumpectomy with radiation and modified radical mastectomy have comparable outcomes."

Getting more African Americans into clinical trials is key to better understanding possible differences in biology. Clinical trial participation has been associated with better survival outcomes. Most national studies into breast cancer are focused on white women and it has only been recently that researchers have started studies to look specifically at black women and other minorities. It takes significant time to build those studies and to get results from them.

Currently, stage II breast cancer outcomes have high five years post-treatment success ratios but my interpretation at the time I was initially diagnosed that I only had five more years period, makes me question so much. I wonder if a white woman who presented the exact same breast cancer would have been given those odds and told the same fate.

CHAPTER 16

STOP THE SILENCE

"What lies behind us and what lies before us are tiny matters compared to what lies within us."
-Oliver Wendell Holmes

alking to a newly diagnosed breast cancer patient takes time and patience. Very few physicians or medical practitioners take the necessary time to thoroughly walk the patient through their pathology report. The report is not in laymen's terms and almost looks foreign. The report may include:

- Is the breast cancer invasive, non-invasive or both?
- Are there lymph nodes involved?
- What did the hormone receptor test show?
- Where the margins negative, positive, or close?
- What lab tests were done on the tissue?
- Was the HER-2 test normal or abnormal?

FOR MOST WOMEN, trying to interpret this report is overwhelming. As a patient, you should demand that your test reports be explained to you in language and terms that you understand. The pathology report is critical in identifying your staging and treatment options so take the time to thoroughly review it and ask questions.

"I REMEMBER the conversation like it occurred yesterday. There I was with a three-page pathology report that my doctor's office had faxed to me. Although I am college educated, it looked like Latin to me. The terms were foreign and the severity of the results was not being understood. I was able to immediately get Karen on the line and she spent an hour consoling me, educating me and simply being a valuable resource as I determined my next course of action in battling stage IIIA breast cancer."
-Crystal Brown-Tatum
Fourteen-year survivor

THERE IS SO much information on breast cancer available in the mainstream media but the urban media has been inconsistent with the early detection and breast health awareness messages. For older women, their main source of obtaining news is community newspapers and if there isn't breast health information readily available, they are missing the mark on patient educational opportunities.

I was fifty years old when I was diagnosed in 1993 and I didn't know the first thing about breast cancer despite the fact that 1993 was an integral time in breast cancer treatment and research. Chemotherapy doses during this time were pretty heavy handed and there was less finesse with regard to patient customization. The heavy doses resulted in harsher side effects and the cure was almost as deadly as the cancer.

In the 1980s, lumpectomy with radiation became a widely used treatment for breast cancers that were found early. In 1985, there were randomized clinical trials that showed lumpectomy was as effective as radical mastectomy. I had a lumpectomy, chemotherapy, and radiation.

CMF is named after the initials of the three drugs used - cyclophosphamide, methotrexate, fluorouracil, which is also known as 5FU. And at the time, it felt like someone was saying five "F" you's!

Each drug is administered separately during the CMF treatment. CMF is used in breast cancer that has an over expression of HER2 and while the classic CMF chemotherapy was shown successful in node negative and node positive forms of breast cancer, the dosages were particularly toxic and caused a host of problems in patients undergoing the therapy regimen. Although it mostly phased out in the 90s, CMF is still seen as a viable treatment despite some of the side effects but is not really used anymore unless anthracyclines like Adriamycin and epirubicin cannot be used.

As physicians understanding and behavior of cancer changed, so did their approach to treatment. This coincided with women becoming more proactive in their health care and actively making decisions about their treatments.

At the same time, the emotional aspects of dealing with breast cancer was also becoming a factor in treatment regimens. As women became more proactive, men began to understand how devastating a diagnosis of breast cancer was and how the loss of a breast or both breasts affected a woman emotionally. Doctors had often given little thought to a woman's frame of mind, concentrating only on saving the patient's life with little regard for her mental well-being. Many male doctors saw these women as mere patients but not whole people who may have had emotional attachments to their breasts. Doctors began to understand more and more that breasts were symbols of womanhood. Women not only wanted to live but they still wanted to take pride in their appearance and not be disfigured.

In the 1990s, breast cancer activism came to the forefront. The pink ribbon symbol was born in the 90s and you would be hard pressed to find someone who did not know the meaning of the pink ribbon.

October is national Breast Cancer Awareness Month and provides an opportunity for us to draw attention to the issue and demand action. Millions of people will donate time and money to purchase "pink" products in support of the cause.

I have always believed in utilizing medical experts when it came to my health. In fact, I clearly stated in our second letter in the summer of 1995, that I strongly supported the ACS's previous recommendations of a baseline mammogram at thirty-five and every other year beginning at forty.

Since the 1950s, advances in mammography are credited for raising the five-year survival rate for localized breast cancer (that hasn't spread from its site of origin) from eighty percent to ninety-eight percent. Mammography is now the number one method of breast cancer detection. Digital mammography gained prominence in the early 90s. Before the early 80s, the mammogram was less a diagnostic tool and was used as a tool to further study anomalies that had already been identified. Digital mammography is still not widely available in sectors although it is said to be most effective for younger women with denser breast tissue. Digital mammography offers more detailed images and easier storage for future comparisons, but it's still not available in many areas, especially outside of cities and major teaching hospitals.

For most women, digital is not any more accurate than regular mammography, but it's about four times as expensive and less likely to be covered by insurance.

In 2007, the American Cancer Society began recommending yearly MRIs for women at high risk for breast cancer, but the procedure is expensive and only available in larger cities. Neither ultrasound nor MRI can detect microcalcifications, which sometimes is the only sign of early cancer. Another disadvantage is that the MRI cannot always distinguish cancer from benign (noncancerous) anomalies, resulting in more biopsies.

Imagine throwing a pebble into a body of water. The ripples slowly get larger and larger. A cancer diagnosis has that same ripple effect on a family. It is a quiet murmur that ends in a loud roar. A cancer diagnosis can be physically and emotionally crippling to all involved.

As you navigate through treatment and on your road to healing, learn to prioritize your day and enlist the help of others. Try and conserve your energy as much as possible. Some energy saving suggestions include:

- Prepare larger portions of food and freeze it
- Sit down to bathe as opposed to taking showers
- Complete as many chores as possible while sitting down
- Try to do light to moderate exercise daily
- Establish a normal sleep pattern

DECISIONS about the appropriate treatment for each patient should be made following a multi-disciplinary team meeting and in discussion with patients and caregivers. It is important that everyone involved in the process is aware of these discussions to enable them to ask and answer questions that patients may have and help to ensure a seamless treatment plan for patients.

If you take the time to learn what to expect during chemotherapy, the temporary side effects may not be as traumatic.

Hair loss does not occur with all chemotherapy medications and people may have different reactions, even with the same medications. You may experience complete hair loss, hair thinning, or may not notice any hair loss at all. Hair loss affects our self-esteem and confidence and is not limited to the hair on our head, but includes eyebrows, pubic hair, nostril hair, and arm hair as well. Some coping methods for hair loss include:

- Cutting your hair prior to chemotherapy to get accustomed to the shorter length.
- Shaving your head before it all falls out to avoid the agony of seeing daily clumps.
- Getting fitted for a wig while you still have hair to better match your color and style. If you can't afford a wig, Sisters Network can assist you in locating a program that offers wig assistance.
- Investing in a variety of hats and head coverings.
- Visiting a cosmetologist to help you learn how to draw in eyebrows or apply makeup to draw attention to other facial features.
- Getting emotional support.
- Read positive books and magazines

CHEMOTHERAPY CAN BE VERY UNPLEASANT, so always keep the lines of communication open with your doctor about how and what you are feeling. There are many medications and remedies available to minimize your discomfort and help you tolerate the powerful drugs. Other chemotherapy side effects may include:

- Nausea/vomiting
- Infection
- Bleeding problems

- Loss of appetite
- Neuropathy-tingling or loss of sensation in fingers and toes
- Chills
- Swelling and fluid retention
- Insomnia
- Joint pain
- Gastrointestinal distress
- Fatigue
- Changes in sexual desires

OF COURSE, this is not a complete list but I stress that if you know what to expect and educate yourself, you can endure treatment better. You will hear so many horror stories that you may actually be afraid to begin the chemotherapy.

In the late 1990s, science confirmed that certain variants (mutations) of the genes BRCA1 and BRCA2 cause up to an eighty percent increase in risk for breast cancer. Some women who discover that they are at high risk take the drastic step of removing their breasts, and sometimes their ovaries, in a radical move to avoid the disease.

I am greatly concerned with recommendations by the U.S. Preventive Services Task Force and U.S. mainstream magazine articles that suggest self-breast exams and mammograms prior to the age of fifty are not very useful. The task force includes doctors, nurses, and researchers, and their 2009 recommendations come a quarter of a century after it was recommended that women get yearly mammograms starting at age forty. Additionally, they concluded there wasn't enough evidence to weigh the benefits and the harms of clinical breast exams beyond mammograms in women age forty and older; recommended mammograms every two years for women ages fifty to

KAREN EUBANKS JACKSON

seventy-four; and recommended against teaching breast self-examination.

The recommended change to the initial mammography screening is very alarming, particularly for African American women who have the highest incidence rate of breast cancer before the age of forty. Before the current baseline is raised, we should investigate reducing the initial mammography screening requirements. Some may conclude that this new recommendation can be viewed as systemic injustice.

As an organization, Sisters Network respects the US Preventive Services Task Force, but our organization will continue to support the previous baseline recommendation to have mammograms starting at age forty and younger if there's a family history.

According to the Canadian Cancer Society, they feel that teaching women to do monthly breast self-exams for cancer does not save lives and is removing monthly breast self-exams off its list of recommended practices saying they are a very poor way to detect cancer. I know too many women who have found their lump during a self-breast exam, or during a mammogram prior to age fifty.

Through my work with Sisters Network, I would surmise that approximately one-half of our members discovered their breast cancers through a routine mammogram prior to the age of fifty. These recommendation changes put women at risks; risks which result in preventable deaths.

In any event, women should be more aware of the state of their breasts at all times. Some guidelines or changes to note when examining your breasts include:

- A lump or swelling in the breast or armpit
- Nipple turning inward
- Change in shape or size of the breast
- Dimpling or puckering of the skin

92

- Nipple discharge or skin scaling
- Pain in any area of the breast

ALTHOUGH SISTERS NETWORK aims to address the unique needs of black women, we fully realize that men can and do get breast cancer.

Actor Richard Roundtree of the 1971 cult favorite "Shaft" fame is perhaps the most well-known male breast cancer survivor. His character John Shaft symbolized masculinity and it took a lot of courage for him to speak out about his personal battle with the disease. Like me, he was also diagnosed in 1993.

"The doctor told me, 'You have breast cancer'," recalls Roundtree. "I heard the cancer part first; it was only later that I heard the breast part. I couldn't believe it."

Roundtree found the lump while filming a movie in Costa Rica. He underwent a double mastectomy and chemotherapy. For years after his diagnosis and treatment, he kept quiet about his status as a cancer survivor. It was after his fifth year, that he decided to speak out and raise awareness of the disease in men.

In the early stages of development of Sisters Network, we featured a male breast cancer survivor in our newsletter who shared his story. He was a forty-nine-year-old male from Oklahoma who underwent a radical mastectomy and chemotherapy. Like many men, he ignored the bb pellet sized lump until it grew to the size of a pencil eraser. By the time of his diagnosis, it had spread to the chest perimeter. He likened chemo to Superman's "Kryptonite" and shared how hard hitting the drugs were. But through his whole testimony, he attributed his strength to God and his faith.

The January 2014 Update authored by Diana Zuckerman, Ph.D. and Anna E. Mazzucco, Ph.D. concluded that the U.S. Preventative Services Task Force, an expert group that reviewed the latest research findings, recommended that mammography screening for most women start at age 50 rather than 40, and that the frequency be every two years (instead of annually) through the age of 74.

The Task Force was widely used as a gold standard for determining medical treatment and screening. In this case, they recommended raising the age to 50 more than two years after the American College of Physicians recommended the same thing, and they also recommended that women continue to undergo mammograms until age seventy-five instead of stopping at sixty-nine. The American Cancer Society strongly disagreed and is still recommending annual mammograms for women over forty.

A key reminder: the Task Force recommendation is for screening mammograms. Mammograms are still needed at almost any age if a lump is found. Women at especially high risk may want to start mammograms at age forty or even earlier.

In spring of 2014, I went in for my annual mammogram. Several days later, I received a phone call notifying me that a spot had been identified and that I needed to come back. I was taken aback to be diagnosed with DCIS breast cancer, but I was armed with knowledge and strength to go back down this journey. It had been twenty years since my initial diagnosis. If I had followed the Task Force recommendation, I would not have had a mammogram screening, and had I been negligent in my monthly self-exams, the new tumor may have gone unnoticed and grown and spread over the course of a year. Had I followed this recommendation, my stage 1 may have been a later stage diagnosis.

This is why it is critical that women perform their monthly self-check breast exams. It will be difficult to identify a new breast lump or any breast changes if you aren't doing these regularly. You cannot rely on recommendations or standard guidelines when you are not standard and your cancer will not wait two years to be detected. So many women diagnosed UNDER forty will not be screened because of insurance regulations and Task Force recommendations. We are experiencing an increase in deaths of young women under forty because they will be diagnosed at late or advanced stage. I am sick and tired of seeing young women die from breast cancer because no one was proactive in their well-being and these young women were literally not taking their own health into their own hands.

The bottom line is that annual mammograms help detect breast cancer early and improve the chances that it can be treated successfully. However, like most medical procedures, there are risks as well as benefits.

Scientific advances are often made by fundamentally changing the way that we look at a problem. Remember that two of the most powerful weapons against breast cancer are early detection and clinical trials. Some tumors become resistant to therapy and can adapt to grow independently and spread to other organs. As addressed in previous chapters, there is still a bit of skepticism in the community when you talk about clinical trials but they are instrumental in the development of improved treatments. Getting African-Americans into clinical trials is key to better understanding possible differences in biology and discovering the best treatments.

The statistics centering on breast cancer can be frightening. It's normal to be afraid, but I challenge you to face those fears head on so that you can address and conquer those fears. Fear can equate to death and breast cancer doesn't have to mean an immediate death sentence.

Some people are born to lead. Others are groomed to become great leaders. I never would have imagined that I would make a career out of breast cancer, but my work with Sisters Network is an extension of my desire to help women feel good about themselves. One of the reasons I pursued jobs in social work and the hair industry is because I enjoyed working with others and helping them. I want to turn each breast cancer diagnosis into a celebration of life.

From day one, my mission was to increase national attention to the devastating impact that breast cancer has in the African American community. Without this attention, our mothers, grandmothers, aunts, cousins, and, of course, sisters will die and their voices silenced forever. The passion and commitment I have for educating my sisters around the world is genuine and unwavering. The statistics are telling our story for us. By educating women before they get breast cancer, they will have good preventive care in place and have a head start on a full recovery should they ever be faced with a diagnosis.

Remember to have a plan of action. Dedicate specific time to mapping out your course of action and asking for help as you navigate through treatment with your medical staff. Develop a resource list and appoint family, friends and supporters to help you with tasks and responsibilities so that you can focus on healing.

CHAPTER 17

SISTERS WALK

*"Divide each difficulty into as many parts as is feasible and necessary
to resolve it and watch the whole transform."*
– Rene Descartes

*P*art of what I discovered in the holistic journey to surviving with breast cancer, was how utterly critical exercise was to my healing. One of the best forms of exercise is walking.

There's no question that walking is good for you. A University of Tennessee study found walking lowers the risk of blood clots, since the calf acts as a venous pump, contracting and pumping blood from the feet and legs back to the heart, reducing the load on the heart.

Walking is a form of exercise that can significantly improve your physical and mental health. Not only can it extend your life and prevent additional disease, but it can also boost your energy and mood.

So if you're one of the 47% of adults in the US who don't meet the CDC's Physical Activity Guidelines for aerobic activity, then walking is a habit worth pursuing and keeping.

In addition to burning calories, walking increases blood flow around the body so that more blood — containing oxygen and nutrients for fuel — can reach the large muscles in the legs as well as the brain. This is what makes you feel energized.

What intrigued me most was discovering that physical exercise like walking increases the amount of white blood cells circulating in your blood. These cells fight infection and other diseases as part of the body's immune system.

In addition, according to studies, walking can increase levels of certain types of chemicals in your brain — known scientifically as neurotransmitters — which help your nervous system work effectively. This can include a type of neurotransmitter that reduces pain.

A study published in the journal *Cancer Epidemiology, Biomarkers, and Prevention*, found that getting out for a walk a few hours a week might help lower your breast cancer risk. Researchers from the American Cancer Society looked at breast cancer status and exercise in nearly 74,000 postmenopausal women. During the 17-year study, 4,760 of the women were diagnosed with breast cancer. Among women whose only physical activity was walking, those who walked seven hours a week had a 14% lower risk for breast cancer compared with those who walked three or fewer hours a week. The longer women walked, and the more strenuously, the lower their risk dropped. It's not clear exactly how exercise might reduce breast cancer risk, but researchers say physical activity helps regulate hormones like estrogen, which can fuel breast cancer growth.

Over the course of our existence, I started feeling like we needed some type of national outreach. I thought a national walk would be great to have that outreach and keep our members healthy. So, in April 2010, Sisters Network, Inc. decided to host our first Stop the Silence 5K Walk/Run in Houston. It was the first national African American walk for breast cancer.

We named our event the Stop the Silence® 5k Walk/Run because of the long-standing history of African Americans not discussing cancer and other life-threatening health concerns. Black women just don't talk enough about this disease that is killing us at a 42 percent higher rate than white women. A recent study conducted by the Ad Council identified that though 92 percent of black women agree breast health is important, only 25 percent of women have recently discussed it, and a mere 17 percent have taken steps to understand their risk.

The walk isn't just about promoting our own health. We walk with a purpose. Proceeds from our walk fund our Sisters Network Breast Cancer Assistance Program. Our walk has raised nearly $1 million in funding to help our sisters.

This national breast cancer walk meant so much to me because we started off as a small group of volunteers knocking door to door and then we had thousands of supporters, black and white, who came out on a rainy Saturday morning and presented a united front in the war against breast cancer.

Our celebrity co-chairs included tennis superstar, Zina Garrison, and television Judge Glenda Hatchett. Legislative and city officials were also in attendance to commemorate this special event.

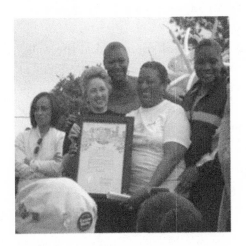

(l to r) Judge Glenda Hatchett, Houston Mayor Anise Parker, Councilwoman Jolanda Jones and Zina Garrison

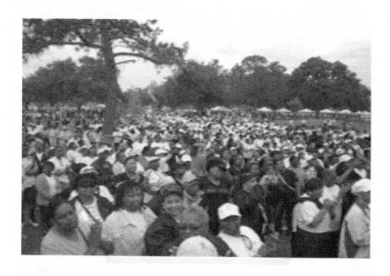

I'm proud that we have been able to gather more than 7,500 people to walk and run and raise money for this cause. Our walk is a beautiful celebration of life. We bring our community together, bring awareness and education about breast cancer and celebrate survivorship. Our sisters come from across the country with their caregivers, family members and friends to show the community what a real sisterhood is all about. Though we can't solve every problem, we know that our BCAP funding can give at least a little relief to our sisters who have so much on their plate when fighting this disease.

"I love seeing the camaraderie and sisterhood at the walk," said Zelma Watkins, co-founder and former vice president of the Central Virginia Affiliate Chapter. "I've walked in all except one, and I always feel good about the unity I see among the survivors, their families and the support of many others who come out to support our survivor community and Sisters Network overall."

The walk is a perfect example of our Sisters Network creed: **'In unity there is strength, in strength there is power, in power there is change.'**

People come from near and far to support our walk—some in busloads, many from church groups—and our sister organization partners The Links, Incorporated, Delta Sigma Theta Sorority, Incorporated and Alpha Kappa Alpha Sorority, Incorporated. We have a special tent where survivors can mingle, hug, share stories, share information and celebrate survivorship. We know the healing power of sisterhood is invaluable.

WHEN I THINK about the turnout at our walks, sometimes I can't help but reflect on that very first Sisters Network meeting at Riverside Clinic.

Today, chapter monthly meetings have thirty to forty regular participants and feature guest speakers on medical aspects of the disease. The stigmas of breast cancer in underserved communities can often leave survivors with a feeling of isolation. Our local chapters provide breast cancer survivors a safe and supportive environment where they can openly address their fears, feelings and concerns. Sisters Network provides unconditional acceptance the moment a survivor joins our family.

A positive attitude can accomplish many tasks. I was simply a woman who had battled breast cancer, who identified a need and developed my vision. Today, Sisters Network Inc. continues to be a leading voice and the only national African American breast cancer survivorship organization in the United States. Our members have served on advisory boards for Susan G. Komen for the Cure, National Cancer Institute and the American Cancer Society and so many others. During 2008, SNI breast health outreach initiatives impacted an estimated 3.6 million families.

The walk helps us refocus on our mission.

People always ask me where the idea for the walk came

from. The answer is simple: From my vision, from my dreams, from my perspective of what's needed to keep us moving forward.

I get these revelations. Some people would say they are messages from God. I haven't determined how these events come or why, but each time I received this message that I should do a certain thing, I actually just start doing it. I don't question it or anything. It puts me in the action mode. And of course, once I feel that I have something positive and complete version of the project, then I present it to the board. The initial part is me just saying, "**Yes, I can.**"

That first walk was a resounding success. And when people ask me why, all I can say is I listened to my intuition and I take action when I feel it. One could say I'm simply projected into action without question. And so far, it's paid off.

In actuality, the same thing happens to me with my physical health situation. My body directs me as to what's wrong and I'm paying attention. And I found all four cancers because I paid attention and listened and took action. Because sometimes you can listen to your body, but you don't take the action.

One of the things I love about the walk is the wonderful spirit of support. It's an amazing sight to see. The walk itself does give our organization visibility within the community. It attracts media and social media and TV and all that helps to promote who you are and what you do.

Attendees are able to interact with others and connect with new people. I love seeing how seriously people take the event. And for survivors who do not have a connection in the city that they are in, it's wonderful to watch them network with other survivors from different parts of the country.

The walk is a sisterhood event that is very positive for our community. And it's a way to raise funds as it doesn't cost much to participate. So, it attracts all people of all types because it's an inexpensive way to help a cause that you believe in.

We see from the registration that not only is it a success, but people love it. They come back year after year and when we had to miss one year, I got a lot of not-so-nice calls and emails asking what happened.

And each year, the walk changes. I look at change as progress, as a movement, as an organization. We're looking for change to improve our circumstances to work on things that haven't changed, to put emphasis on what needs to be done.

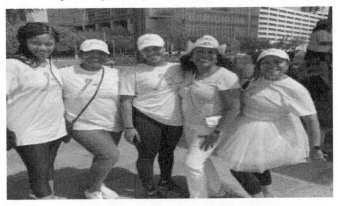

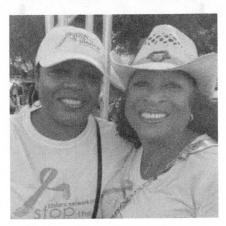

Our walk actually brings joy to the city because it's an expression of thousands of African American people from all of the country who come together. In 10 years, we have never had a negative incident of any kind and I'm very proud of that. It's such a positive experience. You can feel it in the air. You can actually feel the camaraderie and the sisterhood of the participants just by being in the crowd.

Unfortunately, in 2020, the Coronavirus pandemic altered our tenth annual walk. We felt that safety was very important to our membership and because of our physical condition, we didn't need to add an extra problem or risk exposure to COVID-19. We canceled it because it was necessary to keep everyone safe. But I'm confident we'll be back, bigger and better than ever!

CHAPTER 18

WEATHERING STORMS

*"Once the storm is over, you won't remember how you made it
through, how you managed to survive. You won't even be sure, whether
the storm is really over. But one thing is certain. When you come out
of the storm, you won't be the same person who walked in. That's what
this storm's all about.*
-Haruki Murakami

For all the successes that we've had, Sisters Network
has not been without its challenges. But just as we
tackle the disease that ravages our bodies, we forge ahead.

I'm so proud of the work that we do, but it is so unfair to our
community that we're the ones who are leading the way for
African American women and breast cancer. We should not
have to fight every year for the funding to keep the doors open.
And we should not have to fight for our community to support
us, especially in a way that it takes for us to have the movement
be successful.

I find that most people, unless they personally have been
touched by breast cancer, either themselves, a family member, a

friend or a colleague, simply don't take it seriously. And most women don't put our health first. We have a hashtag at SNI: #MakeHealthATopPriority. And we, as a people, are not doing that in general.

When we started, people barely wanted to hear anything about breast cancer. Now they at least open the door but we're still not at the point where the connection is instant.

I wish that I could continue on forever, but again – I listen to my body. And for the last year and a half, I realized I'm getting older and that it's time for me to slow down because of my general physical condition.

Being CEO of Sisters Network every day is a gift but challenging. It's very fast moving and requires constant travel. I've been doing it, but I know that I can't continue. So I've been looking for a replacement so that SNI can go on. The legacy will live on until we find a cure and beyond.

I'm at the point where I think I found the person who should replace me and we're still in a transition period. I'm hoping and praying that the organization will continue to grow and grow even faster and be more impactful.

The movement permeates in multiple cities because when I started this, I felt we needed a Sisters Network in every city. We're well on our way, but we still have a long way to go to be able to reach the women in our community with the message of hope, information and resources and to let them know that they can survive breast cancer.

That move to multiple cities is perhaps one of the most challenging aspects of our goals. There was one point when we had as many as 40 cities under Sisters Network and for different reasons (everything from not meeting membership requirements to leaders passing away) the chapters dissipated. There have been some ups and downs with maintaining and growing chapters in the different communities because each community is different. There's no one shoe that fits all, but we have to make sure that we find the right group of black women in the community who will be responsible for getting the message out and for helping the sisters in their area. That's the advantage of having affiliate chapters. The boots on the ground are very much needed in every city.

My days are full and busy. Between responding to calls and emails, developing new projects, doing webinars, connecting with the different chapters, trying to find funding, writing grants, working on the walk...I stay busy.

And of course, I can't forget, keeping up with the latest information on what's going on in breast cancer research. It's a daily chore, especially in research and development because that's an entity that keeps changing. And I believe that social organizations and community groups have to stay actively involved both locally and nationally.

I'm a proud member of Alpha Kappa Alpha Sorority, Incorporated, which is a very productive sorority, as well as The Houston Chapter of the Links, Incorporated, an outstanding national organization where you have to stay involved in all aspects, which is difficult.

It's my vision to have a national partnership with all black organizations.

Sisters has a relationship with Delta Sigma Theta, Sorority, Incorporated, another nationally known Black sorority. I nurture all these relationships because we overlap with helping each other and that's been very positive. But we need to do more, we need to connect with more organizations and that takes time and effort to really make a difference.

The existence of Sisters Network has helped thousands of women to be able to pick up the phone, call a toll-free number and connect to someone who has the same experience, has a similar background and will take the time to walk you through your journey. That's who we are.

A recent trip to San Antonio summed up why we do what

we do at Sisters Network. I was at an International conference on breast cancer. It's the largest one in the world. As I was going to a dinner, a woman jumped up and stopped me.

"Oh, my, goodness! Karen Jackson. You are my hero." Then, she threw her arms around me and hugged me tightly.

I'd never met this woman but I was happy to greet her with a smile as she continued holding back tears.

"Ten years ago, I was diagnosed with breast cancer. I didn't want to go on. Sisters Network gave me the courage to keep going. And it did so much for me that it inspired me to even start a local group of my own!"

I hugged the woman again, feeling every bit of gratitude in her touch of true sisterhood.

I walked away from that dinner with a smile on my face, feeling inspired once again. Because that's what this is all about: Giving women the strength and the courage to go on and take action.

I always want women to know that there is hope. Get over the initial shock and fear of the words "breast cancer" and get on with living. I personally know many long-term survivors. I am a 27-year survivor; one of our members is a 15-year triple-negative survivor.

There is hope. I believe in living life to the fullest each day in being passionate, productive in every way and making life better for others.

I live my life by 2 Corinthians 5:7: *Walk by faith and not by sight.*

We must start making our health and the quality of health-care we receive a top priority. We tend to misappropriate funds on things we don't really need (hair weave, shoes, purses, fancy cars) and then frown on medical co-pays or out of pocket diagnostic tests.

Breast cancer is a negative situation that I turned into a positive one in my life. I encourage you to do the same with any challenges that may come your way. Find people who believe in you and who support you. You should always be aware of where you can be most helpful.

SNI National Creed

In unity,
there is strength.
In strength,
there is power.
In power,
there is change.

Stop the Silence

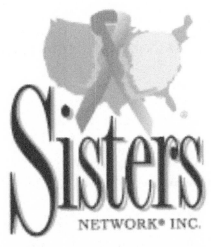

Sisters

NETWORK® INC.

A NATIONAL AFRICAN AMERICAN BREAST CANCER
SURVIVORSHIP ORGANIZATION

CHAPTER 19

STATE OF BLACK BREAST CANCER 2020

#BlackBreastCancer Matters
#SystemicRacismIsTiedToCancer

*O*ne thing that has not changed since I began this breast cancer journey. Breast cancer is the most FATAL health issue for African American Women.

The facts are clear:

- Black women are 42% more like to die of breast cancer
- Black women account for: 12.5% of all new breast cancer cases; 15.5% of all breast cancer deaths
- Black women under 35 get breast cancer at *two times* the rate of white women and die at *three times* the rate.
- The 5-Year Survival rate is: 81% for black women
- vs 91% for white women.
- Black women are often at a more advanced stage upon diagnosis.
- Black breast cancer survivors have a 39% higher risk of breast cancer recurrence.

- Black women have a 2.3 times higher odds of being diagnosed with Triple Negative Breast Cancer.
- Women under age 40 have twice the odds of being diagnosed with triple-negative breast cancer than women aged 50-64 years.
- Among women who were diagnosed with breast cancer, those diagnosed at late stages were 69% more likely to have triple-negative cancer than other types.
- 77.3% of African American moms are single moms.
- 70.5% of all African American working mothers are single moms, making them the primary, if not sole, economic providers for their families.

HERE ARE some more facts worth noting:

- Not only is breast cancer more biologically aggressive in African American women, the disparity in breast cancer mortality also reflects social barriers that disproportionately affect Black women.
- African Americans are significantly underrepresented in clinical research.
- African Americans represent 13.4% of the U.S. population, yet FDA reports that those populations make up only 5% of clinical trial participants.
- Since 2016, the FDA has approved four novel drugs for breast cancer. However, none of those clinical trials had more than 3% black participants.
- A 2014 study indicated that Black women experience emotional suppression and behavioral disengagement — experienced increased levels of distress and poorer survival.

- Black women lack the space to talk about their concerns.
- Black women fear sharing their diagnosis within their families and communities because they are often the family breadwinner.

FACTS ABOUT MOST CANCERS:

I could go on and on. The news about cancer is good for now, but the future doesn't look as bright, according to a report by the American Association for Cancer Research (AACR).

The AACR Cancer Progress Report 2020 found the number of cancer survivors living in the United States has reached a record high, with more than 16.9 million survivors, according to the report.

The U.S. cancer death rate fell by 29% from 1991 to 2017. That's about 2.9 million lives saved, the report said.

Since August 2019, the U.S. Food and Drug Administration has also approved a record number of treatments. Thirty-five were approved between August 2019 and July 31 of this year, several of the treatments are for cancer types that have not had many, or any, options.

The pandemic has taken a toll, having a negative impact on cancer care. Nearly 80% of people in treatment for cancer have experienced some delay in care due to the pandemic.

Looking at data from 190 hospitals in 23 states, the AACR report also found that a number of tests to screen for cervical, breast and colon cancer fell by 85% or more after the first COVID-19 cases was diagnosed in the U.S.

Delays in cancer screenings and treatment are projected to lead to more than 10,000 additional deaths from breast and colorectal cancer over the next decade.

Breast Cancer has not stopped because of COVID-19. Our sisters still need chemo, surgery, scans, bloodwork and are participating in clinical trials. Black women are still being diagnosed with breast cancer on a daily basis requiring screening and treatment. COVID-19 has added a very dangerous layer of complexity to getting critical health care for our Sister Warriors. Add to that how this coronavirus pandemic is disproportionately impacting African Americans. Add to that the number of our Sisters who have lost their jobs and health insurance.

New data also shows that systemic racism is tied to cancer. Great racial disparities remain in cancer survival rates for children and adults.

AACR called for additional consistent government funding for cancer research and better access to health care and screenings.

Scientists also said that individuals can also help themselves and reduce their cancer risk. Regular checkups and timely screenings can detect cancer when it is at a stage where treatment is most effective.

While cancer treatments have improved dramatically over the last several decades, many cancer types still defy standard treatments, including triple-negative breast cancer.

Sisters Network Inc. now participates in #GivingTuesday-Now, a global day of unity and giving. On this Giving Tuesday Now, we seek support for our Breast Cancer Warrior Sisters.

We are truly in unprecedented times and we are all being challenged. Imagine having to deal with all of this with a cancer diagnosis. That's why our work must continue.

In reviewing the past 25 years, we are definitely seeing some proactive changes within our communities and action is now beginning to be a part of who we are. This is a new phenomenon for the black community when it comes to breast cancer. The changing dynamics of life is changing how we tackle breast cancer.

People would turn around and run if you brought up breast cancer in the early years. In 2020, with Black Lives Matter, with the COVID pandemic, people are more in tune with health. As an organization we've always devoted our full attention to put survivors first. Information is power and power changes the trajectory of your journey. #Liveyourlifewithpurpose

Breast cancer does not discriminate so if you don't have it in your family, that does not mean you won't have it. Each of us should have our yearly check-up. You could be the first one in your family. Most of us don't know our family history anyway, so we must be proactive.

Another aspect we're now including is mental health, which was never a component of the discussion or research when it came to breast cancer. In retrospect, it should've always been a part of the conversation. The systematic injustices that have always existed, affects us mentally, and therefore should now and forever more, be included in who we are how we respond to medical issues.

I wish I had known to include mental health in the very beginning. It affects all of us, but we didn't look at mental health in a scientific way. It's a critical part that was omitted.

Not anymore. Mental health is important. Education is ever-evolving and a key component to winning this battle against breast cancer. #FindingaNewNormal.

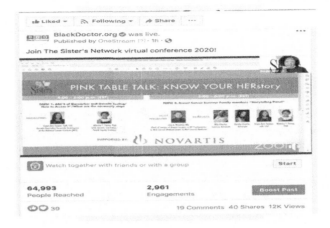

Like many organizations, Sister's Network has had to figure out how adapt to the new normal by hosting virtual events.

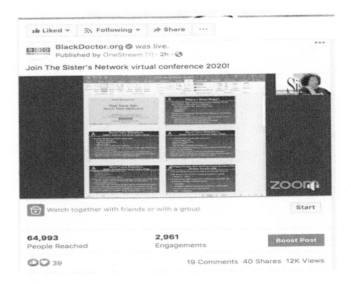

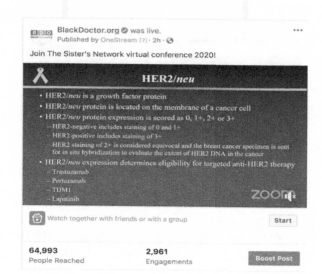

BlackDoctor.org ✅ was live.
Published by OneStream [?] · 2h · 🌐

Join The Sister's Network virtual conference 2020!

HER2/*neu*

- HER2/*neu* is a growth factor protein
- HER2/*neu* protein is located on the membrane of a cancer cell
- HER2/*neu* protein expression is scored as 0, 1+, 2+ or 3+
  - HER2-negative includes staining of 0 and 1+
  - HER2-positive includes staining of 3+
  - HER2 staining of 2+ is considered equivocal and the breast cancer specimen is sent for in situ hybridization to evaluate the extent of HER2 DNA in the cancer
- HER2/*neu* expression determines eligibility for targeted anti-HER2 therapy
  - Trastuzumab
  - Pertuzumab
  - TDM1
  - Lapatinib

ZOOM

📦 Watch together with friends or with a group   Start

64,993
People Reached

2,961
Engagements

Boost Post

CHAPTER 20

YOU ARE NOT ALONE - SURVIVOR STORIES

NORA JONES

MY BREAST CANCER STORY

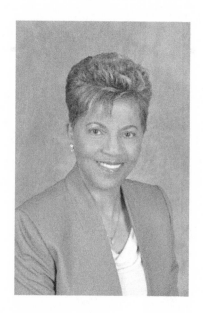

*I*n July 2007, I went in for my yearly mammogram. Although my sister died of breast cancer at age 54 in 1992, I was not too concerned about the genetic risk. In fact, breast cancer was the farthest thing from my mind on that day.

Consequently, I was shocked to learn of my diagnosis of DCIS, ductal carcinoma in situ. I was handed a notebook of cancer resources and a manual on breast cancer. Then, the radiologist wished me good luck and said good-bye. I was struck by the cold, matter-of-fact way the diagnosis was communicated. That was the one day I truly craved some compassion and warmth, instead I felt alone, helpless and filled with anxiety.

In the meantime, I called the local office of the American Cancer Society about getting a mentor. I received the name and phone number of a breast cancer survivor who was willing to answer general questions I had. However, I wanted an African American mentor, and there was none available at the time. The ACS referred me to Sisters Network. I eventually ended up calling Valarie Worthy in Durham and Jamie Gaston of Charlotte. These two ladies were there for me when I needed them most. I am truly indebted to them for their kindness and encouragement. Because of them, I became more determined than ever to establish a Sisters Network chapter in Greensboro.

The recommended treatment for my diagnosis was a lumpectomy followed by six weeks of radiation to the right breast. My quality of life was reduced to going to radiation therapy and returning home to remain in bed for the rest of the day. Finally, the oncologist recommended that I take "bee pollen tablets" to raise my energy level, and they worked! I felt so much better and I was able to get out more. In addition, another friend recommended acupuncture. I was skeptical at first, but I did try one acupuncture session. I was amazed at how wonderful I felt.

Currently, I am a breast cancer survivor of twelve years. I feel great, and although I experience minor health problems from time to time, I consider myself to be truly blessed.

BETTIE K. EUBANKS

FRIENDS 'TIL THE END

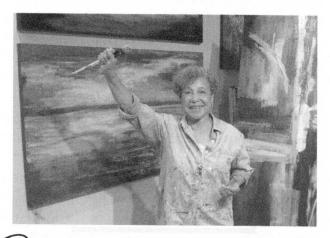

A childhood friendships that's lasted a lifetime... That's who and what we are.

Karen and I met in church as young girls. From Sunday school through high school, we giggled, we laughed and we talked. We talked about everything. Once we were so involved in our conversation, we never noticed the school bus just rolled right past us and we had to run to school. There has never been a time when we could not talk about any and every subject and so when Karen had a calling to support our African American sisters in their walk with breast cancer, we continued to talk and I continued to listen and support Karen in her efforts. And thus, was born Sisters Network Inc, (SNI) was born.

Sisters Network Inc. grew out of a need in the United States that was not supported by any other breast cancer organization for our African American sisters.

My support of Karen's breast cancer pledge grew from an idea in her apartment to my support as a member of the board of SNI for over 10 years. Our conversations of women being able to discuss their concerns and being supported by the camaraderie of conversation and education grew into an idea for the logo art piece "Sisters." The original art piece was given to Karen. A lithograph was printed from the original art piece, which I signed and donated to SNI with 100% of the proceeds donated to the organization. The women in the organization identified with the subject in the lithograph and all 250 of the art pieces now reside in the homes and offices of the members and supporters of SNI.

Our friendship continues to be a wonderful journey. Now that I, too, am a breast cancer survivor, Karen's conversations and support have taken on one more valuable dimension. We still laugh and talk about anything and everything. We continue to share and enjoy each other as friends and family. What we have is sisterhood, it is friendship and bottom line it's love of a friend.

DIANNE TOWNSEND

INSPIRED TO SUPPORT

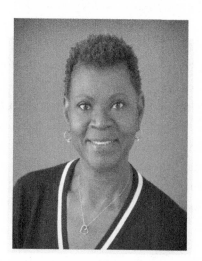

*I*n August 1997, I helped establish Sisters Network Northeast Florida in Jacksonville, FL, where I have served as Chapter President since its inception. After my own diagnosis of an ER+ breast cancer in 1987, I began to learn about the disease and began to advocate for myself.

However, after meeting Karen in Houston in April 1997, I became committed to encouraging and supporting other survivors to grow the chapter back home.

Connecting with other African American survivors through both Sisters Network Inc. and the new local chapter was an immense help in gaining control of a devastating diagnosis during a time when little survivorship support was available in the community. Furthermore, in the twenty-three years as President of Northeast Florida Chapter, thousands of women in Jacksonville have benefited from the cancer education, screening, and awareness initiatives of Sisters Network Inc.

Thankful to God for thirty-three years of survivorship, including several recurrences, I continue to serve as Chapter President, advocating, motivating, educating, and assisting other breast cancer survivors in understanding this disease and its effects on the African American community.

SHAWNTELL MCWILLIAMS

A NEW BEGINNING

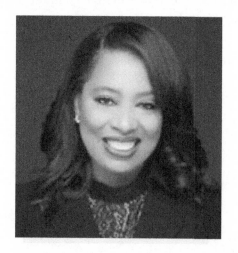

*T*he year was 2012. It was the start of a new chapter for me. I had just moved to Houston, Texas from Shreveport, Louisiana and married the love of my life, Keith McWilliams. Everything was falling into place and I was living my best life until my worst fear came to pass.

While going through my daily routine, I felt a lump on my breast wall; instantly, I thought it was my worst fear - breast cancer. Even still, I have to admit that I was in denial and ignored it (at least I tried).

After a conversation with my mother and sister, I scheduled a mammogram at MD Anderson. It was there that I received the devastating diagnosis of Stage IIIB triple positive, HER2 positive breast cancer.

I was 37 years old.

A newlywed for two months and new resident of Houston, I was scared, and bombarded with feelings of defeat. There was no family history or breast cancer, and no blueprint on how to fight this disease. So I began to isolate myself and mentally and emotionally withdraw.

My sister reached out to Sisters Network, Inc. Eventually, I forged a close friendship with Karen Jackson. She became influential during my breast cancer journey. Karen's story of survivorship was inspirational to me and displayed an African American woman who beat breast cancer and was thriving fabulously!

I underwent six months of chemotherapy, which was conducted weekly; six weeks of radiation therapy; a year of Herceptin (another type of chemotherapy to treat HER2 positive breast cancer); and three surgeries. The treatments took a toll on my body. I developed blood clots and was diagnosed with polymyositis (an autoimmune condition that breaks down your muscles).

At one point during my journey in defeating breast cancer, I found it difficult to walk or stand on my own without assistance that resulted from the polymyositis. In those lowest moments, and you will have them, I found three things that helped me cope – the support system of my family and friends, writing a journal of my feelings, and staying spiritually fed by listening to Gospel recording artist Marvin Sapp.

After completing my intense breast cancer treatments, I joined Sisters Network as Vice President for two years. My passion is in serving others and giving back to my community, as well as assisting other survivors with their breast cancer

journey through strategic partnerships, national program operations, and fundraising.

I have devoted my life to serving others through my phil-
anthropic efforts, spending time with my family/friends, and
working alongside my husband, Keith, in our businesses.

JANICE E. WORKCUFF

FACING REALITY

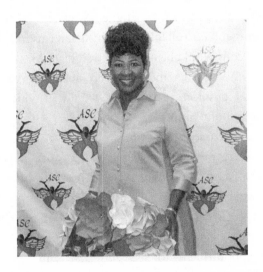

*A*bout the middle of February 1988, I was wrestling with my 5-year-old son, William, Jr. I was trying to grab his hand and it slipped and he accidentally hit my left breast, sending a very painful blow. As I grabbed my breast with the palm of my hand, it rested on a lump.

I always performed my monthly breast examination, and I had never noticed this before. I had never had a mammogram before because all the information I had read stated that your first mammogram was to be done at age forty. I was only thirty-two years of age. I had a mammography. The physician then proceeded to read my report:

"An ill-defined, somewhat lobulated density, approximately 2.5 cm in the outer left quadrant of the left breast, close to the chest wall. Biopsy may be appropriate. If biopsy is not appropriate, repeat mammogram in six months." I was not comfortable waiting six months. I made an appointment with another physician that same day. He agreed with me that the only sure way of ruling out malignancy was to perform an open incision biopsy surgical removal with the microscopic examination of the suspicious tissue. The physician gave me a sense of comfort. The biopsy was positive for malignancy (cancer) of the breast. I started crying uncontrollably. The physician carefully explained our next options would be a Modified Radical Mastectomy, or a lumpectomy. I was ERA and PRA were negative. We decided to get a second opinion, feeling this would provide us with a certain amount of comfort.

After we discussed the options, I decided to have a modified radical mastectomy. The surgeon had informed me that the cancer was caught in time. About three months after the surgery, I woke up with a feeling of fullness in my chest. When I looked in the mirror, I noticed that the area on my chest where the mastectomy had been was red and slightly protruding. I made an appointment to see him that same morning. He proceeded to tell me that the fullness in my chest was because of a manifestation of cancer cells. Evidently, a group of cancer cells must have broken away from the original tumor and migrated through the lymph system and blood stream. These cells had started growing. I was having a recurrence. It was recommended that I undergo toxic chemotherapy and my physician wanted me start immediately. He explained all the side effects. I would have the chemotherapy twice a week. These treatments would be a strong preventative measure. Cytoxan, 5-FU (fluorouracil), and Adriamycin were the chemotherapy drugs I would be receiving. After this treatment, I would begin having radiation therapy treatments, which I would receive twice a day for six weeks.

This was all moving so fast. But I kept remembering "God is not of fear." I kept a positive attitude During the third chemotherapy treatment, my hair started to fall out and I was devastated – another loss. After the radiation, I went in for another series of tests to detect if there was any more evidence of cancer cells anywhere else in my body. Thankfully, the results all came back negative. **"ON A MISSION NOT REMISSION"**

It's been 32 years and I am grateful, and I stand in the gap for others on this breast cancer journey.

Janice is former President of Sisters Network Affiliate Houston Chapter, Executive director of Angels Surviving Cancer, Inc.

ZELMA C. WATKINS

FIGHTING A GOOD FIGHT

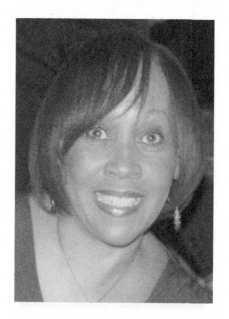

*A*t the age of 44, a routine mammogram eventually led to a shocking diagnosis of triple negative breast cancer. I underwent intensive chemotherapy and radiation after having a lumpectomy, I am currently celebrating twenty years as a breast cancer survivor.

It was this journey with breast cancer that led me to Sisters

Network Inc. At the time of my diagnosis, I didn't know anyone with breast cancer, nor did I know anything about it. Frankly, I was surprised with my diagnosis as there was no history of breast cancer in my family — at least, nothing that was discussed. But more disturbing, there were so few resources for women of color at the time.

Since joining Sisters Network in 2000, I have been a dedicated and active member of the organization and have held several positions, including: member, National Advisory Council (NAC); Co-Chair, 6ᵗʰ Annual National Conference in Richmond, VA; Secretary, Sisters Network Inc. Board of Directors; and National Director, Young Sisters Initiative (YSI). In addition, I served as a Sisters Network liaison with the Center for Disease and Control.

I am determined to create awareness about breast cancer and to help ensure breast cancer is not a death sentence for African American women in the Richmond Metro area. That's why I co-founded the first Sisters Network affiliate chapter in Richmond, Virginia in October 2001, and in 2005, and became the founder of a second Richmond-based affiliate chapter, Sisters Network Central Virginia Inc.

In 2012, the chapter was presented with the "Trail Blazer Award" for outstanding community service during the organization's 13ᵗʰ Annual Leadership Conference in Houston, TX.

Through my work with Sisters Network and other advocacy efforts, I have developed several alliances within the Richmond community. I have served on the Breast & Cervical Cancer Early Detection Review Committee, as well as the advisory board for The Ellen Shaw de Parades Breast Cancer Foundation. I currently serve on the Board for Reach Out for Life.

While my breast cancer diagnosis was life changing, I am fortunate to not only be alive, but to be positioned to share my testimony and help create awareness about the devastating impact breast cancer has in the African American community.

KAREN EUBANKS JACKSON

Beyond my advocacy work, I am active in my community. I retired from the United Parcel Service (UPS) after 34 years of service. Before my retirement, I served as a Strategic Account Sales Manager for the East Central Region. Training people and seeing them develop to their full potential was one of the best aspects of my job. I took that same passion and applied it to volunteer efforts mentoring middle school girls through the Mega Mentors program. I also volunteer with the Basic Blessing Clothing Ministry of her church—First Baptist Church of South Richmond.

When I am not volunteering, I am helping individuals find their dream home as a licensed realtor.

CRYSTAL BROWN TATUM

STILL STANDING

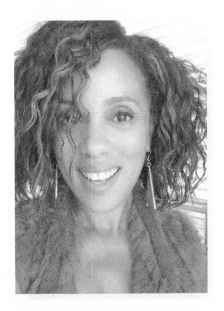

*T*he year was 2007. I was 35, full of life and had just walked down the aisle to marry the man of my dreams when I got the news. I was diagnosed with stage 3A triple negative breast cancer. To say I was devastated and lost would be an understatement.

After feverishly searching the Internet for readily available resources for women of color, I was disappointed, until I remembered that my friend, Caleen's mother was a survivor who started a national breast cancer organization for African American women.

I reached out to Karen, who immediately took my call and stayed on the phone with me for over an hour, providing expert advice, guidance and support. Armed with the knowledge and inspiration from that initial call, I proceeded fearlessly through my aggressive treatments and was led to begin a Sisters Network chapter in Shreveport. After a military relocation out of the area and the death of the chapter Vice President, the chapter dissolved, but not without making a noticeable improvement in community awareness.

I continue my advocacy work with Sisters Network through my ongoing work with PCORI-Patient Centered Outcomes Research Institute in Washington, D.C. As a patient mentor and reviewer, I attend the annual meeting and bring the patient and community voice to the table, where evidence-based research decisions are being made. I also shared my story with my elected officials at the state and national level.

Not one to shy away from accountability, I took full responsibility for my late stage diagnosis and made it my mission to educate others about the importance of early detection. My story has been featured in numerous media outlets, including *Self, Ebony* and *Essence* magazines and I have been a guest on the "Dr. Oz Show." I am the author of "Saltwater Taffy and Red High Heels: My Journey through Breast Cancer," which details my treatment journey from diagnosis to remission. I wrote the memoir when I could not locate a book written by a black author online or in my community. To date, the book has been sold across the globe and I continue to be a sought-out motivational speaker on the topic.

Sisters Network® Inc. has provided so much tangible and

measurable support to my friends and me throughout the years. From bill pay assistance to clinical trial opportunities, the organization has navigated me on my healing journey. I remain grateful to Karen and every sister in the network who provided a sounding board and crutch when I needed it most.

TAMIKO BYRD

FEAR NO MORE

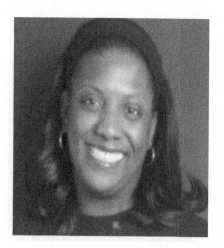

A year after relocating my family to Houston, I participated in a wellness challenge that would lead to the discovery of stage IV breast cancer by Student Health Services of TWU. I went from not so much as taking an aspirin to chemotherapy.

I have to admit - I had extreme fear and anguish. After watching my father and two of my brothers die from pancreatic cancer within five years of each other, and as a divorced mother of three sons, I asked the question, "Who would raise my children?"

I was determined to FIGHT FOR MY LIFE. I learned all I could about breast cancer, specifically, Ductal Carcinoma In Situ (DCIS). Still the diagnosis was devastating! Family and friends were extremely present and supportive, yet I still felt alone with this disease.

As a member of Lilly Grove Missionary Baptist Church, in Houston, I was introduced to members who were breast cancer survivors and learned about Sisters Network and Founder, Karen Jackson. When I was invited to the Pink Sisters Network House in October 2016, I immediately felt at home.

Karen Jackson met personally with me and shared her personal breast cancer journey as well as all the wonderful services that Sisters Network offered, such as the Breast Cancer Assistance Program (BCAP), chapter support groups, and the amazing Stop the Silence walk!

I no longer felt alone in this disease. I had the strength of Sisters Network to fight breast cancer...and beat IT!!! Additionally, I earned dual degrees – a Master of Science in Kinesiology and an Executive MBA in December 2017 while battling stage IV breast cancer.

Today, I am a doctoral student at Southern Nazarene University in Oklahoma. I also own my own independent insurance agency, TEE BYRD INSURANCE, BOOKKEEPING & TAX, servicing over 20 states in the U.S. I am a four-year Breast Cancer Survivor and four-year national volunteer with Sisters Network.

I attribute my survival to the support I received from Sisters Network and Karen Jackson.

"Survive, Serve, Support Sisters Simultaneously" is the phrase that I carry in my heart and is the phrase that saved my life. I vow to share my story and support Sisters Network for the rest of my life!

CECILIA POPE

CHOOSING LIFE

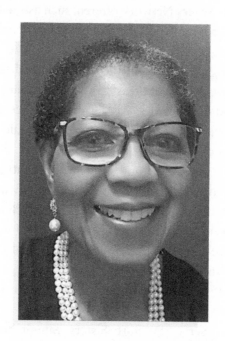

As a retired Pediatric Nurse with over 40 years of experience, I knew all too well the importance of good health and advocating for self-care. I faithfully performed monthly self-breast exams, received yearly physical breast exams by my gynecologist and received my yearly mammogram screening.

Nonetheless, at the age of 45, I found myself facing a devastating health diagnosis of my own, Infiltrating Duct Carcinoma. Even more alarming, was the fact that there was no history of breast cancer in my family, and I did not fit any of the typical risk factors.

Since my diagnosis, one of my biological sisters was diagnosed with breast cancer seven (7) years later. I did have genetic counseling and testing done in 2015. I do not carry the BRCA1 and the BRCA2 genes.

Although a routine mammogram confirmed the breast cancer diagnosis, I actually discovered my area of concern during a shower. It was not a defined lump or tumor that I felt, but an unusual "area of thickness." Not all breast cancers come in the form of lumps and tumors. I had a Lumpectomy, followed by chemotherapy and radiation. I also received adjuvant therapy of Tamoxifen over a five-year period.

I'm happy to say I am currently celebrating life as a 25-year breast cancer survivor.

As part of my journey to healing physically, emotionally and spiritually, I joined a breast cancer support group named "WAVE" (Women Achieving Victory and Esteem). It was through WAVE that a connection to Dr. Lisa Newman MD, Surgical Breast Oncologist, led to the meeting of Karen Eubanks Jackson, Founder & CEO of Sisters Network Inc.

Karen's breast cancer journey, her passionate belief in the need to start a survivorship organization that addressed the unique needs of African American women facing this devastating disease, and the mission of Sisters Network Inc. resonated with the members of WAVE. As a result, a Detroit Chapter of Sisters Network Inc. was formed.

I am one of the founding members of the Sisters Network Greater Metropolitan Detroit Chapter (SNGMDC), which was instituted on August 7, 2001. I have been a loyal, committed and active member since the beginning. I have held various leadership positions from Treasurer, Vice-President, and currently, President. I am very passionate about the mission of Sisters Network Inc. and was very instrumental in developing a local breast cancer brochure specifically for the Detroit Chapter. In addition, I also developed a "talking points" card with important bullet point facts about the Detroit Chapter's history, for members to use as a reference when out and about in the community at speaking engagements.

Breast cancer is a very devastating disease on many levels. For many women it is a personal attack on their femininity. It is viewed as body image destruction/disfigurement. It is a loss of breast tissue, a loss of a breast or both. It is the loss of hair. It is even the loss of life. The diagnosis is truly life-changing. But despite all the negative devastation, I choose to see the positive. I feel truly blessed and thankful to be alive. I feel a deeper appreciation for life, a keener sense of awareness of others' feelings and needs, and a clearer understanding of my life's purpose.

My journey is my story/testimony that I feel compelled to share in order to give a glimmer of hope to someone struggling with the fear of their diagnosis. Breast cancer is not an automatic death sentence. Early detection is the key to survival. Following through on the treatment plan is paramount. Our true beauty is deeper than what is physically on the outside. Beauty radiates from within our heart and our soul.

CALEEN ALLEN

A TRIBUTE TO MY MOTHER

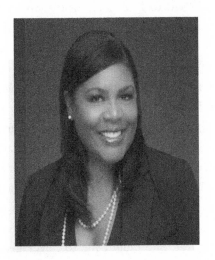

*M*any people know and recognize Karen Eubanks Jackson as a four-time breast cancer survivor, Founder and CEO, Sisters Network Inc., a nationally recognized speaker and breast cancer advocate, and now author of ***In the Company of My Sisters, My Story, My Truth***. To me, she is simply Mom, my hero and best friend.

For the last 27 years, I have had the privilege, honor and a front row seat as I watched her courageously take a personal health challenge and create Sisters Network Inc., the only

National African American breast cancer survivorship organization in the United States to educate and support black women. She is a true visionary whose desire was to build a sisterhood to support black breast cancer survivors, increase awareness in the black community to save lives and mobilize women to take action so they can live their best lives despite battling breast cancer. Karen Eubanks Jackson not only accomplished her mission, but also earned a respected reputation as a pioneer and a legacy as a leading voice in the national Black breast cancer movement.

Not many people find their true purpose and passion, my mother was blessed to find her purpose and passion after her first breast cancer diagnosis in 1993. In her memoir, she chronicles her journey as a young woman from the East Coast, a wife, mother, grandmother, beating breast cancer four-times and founding the nation's largest black breast cancer survivorship organization. *In the Company of My Sisters, My Story, My Truth* is her story about living life on purpose, never losing hope or giving up on yourself, standing in your truth and recognizing the importance of making your health a top priority.

There is no doubt that Karen Eubanks Jackson is a role model and an inspiration to many women around the nation. Her courage and strength are unwavering. She is a survivor and a relentless fighter. She taught me to never give up on life no matter what challenges may come my way.

My mother and I share a love and special bond that can never be broken. I am proud of the legacy she has built as one of the leading national voices in the fight against breast cancer in the black community. Most importantly, I am so proud and blessed that Karen Eubanks Jackson is my mother and forever hero.

A NOTE FROM THE AUTHOR

MY STORY, MY TRUTH

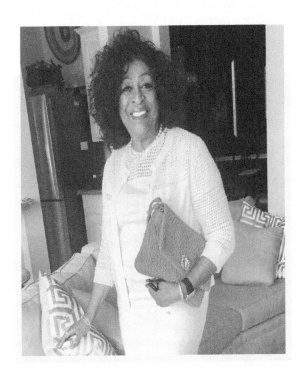

*T*here are so many people in my life that I am grateful for toward that my acknowledgments could be a book in and of itself. I am humbled and grateful by the overwhelming support of Sisters Network® Inc., over the years.

On behalf of Sisters Network Inc.'s Board of Directors, we sincerely appreciate everyone who has lent their time, financial support, or resources to the organization since its inception in 1994. No act of support has been overlooked or is considered too small. To borrow from an African proverb . . . It has taken a village.

Extreme gratitude to my mother, Carliese Mason Eubanks, and father John Scott Eubanks. Although they are no longer physically here, they continue to live in my heart and are a part of my daily life. Thank you for a loving, healthy upbringing that molded me into the woman I am today.

Thank you to my husband, Kyle, of 34 years - my partner for life - for your unconditional love and support. You were always by my side through the good times and the challenging times.

Thank you to my loving, beautiful and talented daughter, Caleen Burton Allen, for being a remarkable inspiration to me and for directly influencing each step of the organization's development.

I'd like to thank the wonderful staff and Board of Directors at National Headquarters over the years for their hard work and dedication to ensuring that the organization stays first class and able to meet the needs of our survivor membership and the black community.

I'd like to thank all of the dedicated affiliate chapter presidents, past and present, and all of the breast cancer survivor members nationwide who continue to work tirelessly toward finding a cure. The organizational growth would not be possible without this dedicated breast cancer survivor base, community volunteers and financial support from pharmaceutical companies, sororities, fraternities, social organizations, churches and businesses.

To several of my longtime special friends who have encouraged me over these many years when Sisters was just an idea: Yvonne Johnson, Judith Chambers, Paula Church. Last but not least, my family, sister-in-law Bettie Kimbro Eubanks, and sister, Kim M. Kirkland.

This book is dedicated to every person whose life has been touched by breast cancer. "**Together**, we must work toward a cure. **Together** we can heal. **Together**, the journey is made easier".

-KEJ

She's not heavy; she's my SISTER.

Visit the author at www.KarenEubanksJackson.com
Contact the author at: info@kareneubanksjackson.com
Visit Sisters Network at www.SistersNetworkInc.org

APPENDIX

Allday, Erin. **"Breast Cancer Mortality Studies in Black Women."** SFGate home of the San Francisco Chronicle. Published May 18, 2007. 9 September 2009.
    <www.sfgate.com/cgibin/article.cgi?
f=/c/a/2007/05/18/BAGEIPTFED1.DTLixzz0SzQjuxTM>.

U.S. Preventive Services Task Force, **Screening for Breast Cancer**: Recommendation Statement, http://www.ahrq.-gov/clinic/uspstf09/breastcancer/brcanrs.htm#update}

American Cancer Society. **"Breast Cancer Facts and Figures 2009-2010."** Atlanta: American Cancer Society, Inc.

American Cancer Society. **"Mammograms and Other Breast Imaging Procedures."**
cancer.org. October 15, 2009.
<http://www.cancer.org/Healthy/FindCancerEarly/
ExamandTestDescr
Mammograms and Other Breast Imaging Procedures/index?
sitearea=PED>.

Armstrong, K., McMurphy, S., Peters, N., Shea, J.A. "**Distrust of Health Care System and Self-Reported Health in the United States.**" Journal of General Internal
Medicine. 2006 Apr, 21(4):292-7.

Arnold, R., Brufsky, A., Rosenzweig, M.Q., Wiehagen, T. "**Challenges of Illness in Metastatic Breast Cancer: A Low-Income African-American Perspective.**"
Palliative and Supportive Care. 2009 v.7:143-152.

Goodwin, Sue. "**American Cultural History, 1940-1949.**" Lone Star College- Kingwood.
Updated July 2009. 4 January 2010 <http://kclibrary.lonestar.edu/decade40.html>.

Huff, Charolette. "**Laymen's Terms: How to Translate the Language of Cancer.**" Cure Magazine. 2009 Winter 8(4):22-5.

King, William D. "**Examining African-Americans' Mistrust of the Health Care System: Expanding the Research Question.**" Public Health Reports. 2003
July-Aug, 118:366-7.

Kinnon, J.B. "**How to Beat Breast Cancer: The Importance of Detecting and Treating Breast Cancer Early.**" findarticles.com- BNET. Ebony, 2010 Sep. 17 November 2009.
<http://findarticles.com/p/articles/mi_m1077/is_12_55/ai_65572098/>. LaTour, Kathy. "**Breast Cancer Around the World.**" Cure Magazine. 2009 Fall 8(3):

LeBrasseur, N., Van Epps, H. L. "**Targeting the Triple Threat.**" Cure Magazine. 2009 Fall 8(3)

Lee-Frye, Betsy. **"How Breast Cancer May Affect Body Image: Scars, Hair Loss, and Weight Gain Are Among the Challenges."** About.com. Updated Dec 05 2008.

Reviewed by site's Medical Review Board. 17 November 2009

<http://breastcancer.about.com/lw/Health-Medicine/Conditions-anddiseases/

How-Breast-Cancer-May-Affect-Body-Image.htm> .

Lerner, Barron. **"History of Breast Cancer Treatment through the Twentieth Century."**

Fresh Air/ WHYY/ NPR 24 May 01. Mindfully.org. 6 October 2009

http://www.mindfully.org/Health/Breast-Cancer-Treatment-History.htm

Maguire, P., Parkes, C. **"Coping with Loss: Surgery and Loss of Body Parts."** British Medical Journal. 1998 Apr 316(7137):1086-88.

"Multicultural Issues and Resources: African-American Women." Breast Cancer Resource Directory of North Carolina and UNC's Lineberger Comprehensive

Cancer Center. 3 February 2010.

<http://bcresourcedirectory.org/directory/05-african_american.htm>.

"The 1940: Lifestyles and Social Trends: Overview." American Decades. 2001.

Encyclopedia.com. 3 Feb 2010 <http://www.encyclopedia.com>.

Tuttle, B.R. "How Newark became Newark: The Rise, Fall and Rebirth of an American

City." Newark, NY. Rutgers University Press, Mar 2009.

"Who was MD Anderson?" The University of Texas MD Anderson Center.
  copyright 2010. 17 November 2009 <http://www.mdanderson.org/about-us/factsand-
    history/who-was-m-d-anderson-/index.html>.

"Your Guide to the Breast cancer Pathology Report." Breastcancer.org.   September   2009.
<http://www.herceptin.com/pdf/pathology_report.pdf>.

Breast Cancer Rates Among Black Women and White Women
  https://www.cdc.gov/cancer/dcpc/research/articles/breast-
  _cancer_rates_women.htm

Cancer Facts & Figures 2020
  https://www.cancer.org/research/cancer-facts-statistics/all-
cancer-facts-figures/cancer-facts-figures-2020.html